KU-505-679

HAMILTON BAILEY'S

# Demonstrations of Physical Signs: Picture Tests

## J.S.P. Lumley MS FRCS

Professor of Surgery
St Bartholomew's Hospital
London, UK

## Shirley Chan FRCS

Specialist Registrar in General Surgery
South East Thames Region
UK

## Heather Harris FRCS

SHO in Urology
St George's Hospital
London, UK

## Mustafa O Mahmoud Zangana FRCS

Honorary Specialist Registrar
Newham General Hospital
London, UK

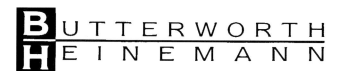

OXFORD   AUCKLAND   BOSTON   JOHANNESBURG   MELBOURNE   NEW DELHI

Butterworth-Heinemann
Linacre House, Jordan Hill, Oxford OX2 8DP
225 Wildwood Avenue, Woburn, MA 01801-2041
A division of Reed Educational and Professional Publishing Ltd

ℛ A member of the Reed Elsevier plc group

First published 2000

Text © Hamilton Bailey (Medical Works) Limited and Reed Educational and
Professional Publishing Ltd 2000
Illustrations © St Bartholomew's Hospital and the Royal School of Medicine and
Dentistry of Queen Mary and Westfield College, London 2000

All rights reserved. No part of this publication may be reproduced in
any material form (including photocopying or storing in any medium by
electronic means and whether or not transiently or incidentally to some
other use of this publication) without the written permission of the
copyright holder except in accordance with the provisions of the Copyright,
Designs and Patents Act 1988 or under the terms of a licence issued by the
Copyright Licensing Agency Ltd, 90 Tottenham Court Road, London,
England W1P 0LP. Applications for the copyright holder's written
permission to reproduce any part of this publication should be addressed
to the publishers

**British Library Cataloguing in Publication Data**
A catalogue record for this book is available from the British Library

**Library of Congress Cataloguing in Publication Data**
A catalogue record for this book is available from the Library of Congress

ISBN 0 7506 4339 0

Composition by Genesis Typesetting, Rochester, Kent
Printed and bound in Great Britain

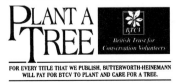

FOR EVERY TITLE THAT WE PUBLISH, BUTTERWORTH-HEINEMANN
WILL PAY FOR BTCV TO PLANT AND CARE FOR A TREE.

(Per Leeds Replacements)

£40.00    14/9/06

NLM    WO
Class    141
Mark:    LUM
Chapel Allerton

HAMILTON BAILEY'S

# Demonstrations of Physical Signs: Picture Tests

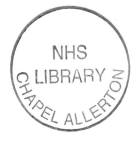

NHS LIBRARY CHAPEL ALLERTON

# Contents

Preface     vii

Questions and Answers     1

Index     193

# Preface

Clinical diagnosis is based on a detailed clinical history, a thorough clinical examination and appropriate investigations: it is greatly facilitated by previous experience of any problem, this being particularly so with visual recall. The repeated exposure to clinical signs, by contact with patients and by illustrative material, reinforces this information gathering.

This text presents illustrations from the 18th edition of *Hamilton Bailey's Demonstrations of Physical Signs in Clinical Surgery**, together with questions about the underlying disease. Illustrations are placed in random order to avoid sequential clues. The answers appear on the reverse of the page of questions and provide details of each condition. For a more comprehensive coverage of these diseases, the reader is referred to the parent volume.

In the early part of their studies, students are advised to use the pictures, questions and answers to acquire useful packages of information. Later, the book provides a means to revise physical signs from across the whole surgical curriculum.

*Lumley, J.S.P. (1997) *Hamilton Bailey's Demonstrations of Physical Signs in Clinical Surgery*, 18th edition, Oxford: Butterworth-Heinemann. ISBN 0 7506 1621 0.

# Questions and answers

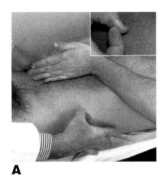

**A**

1 What sign is being demonstrated?

2 What other signs may be demonstrable in this patient?

3 What are the causes of ascites?

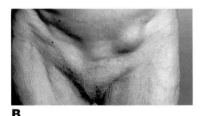

**B**

1 What are these two swellings?

2 How would you differentiate between the swellings?

3 What are the complications of these lesions?

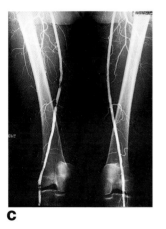

**C**

1 What does this arteriogram show?

2 What symptoms might the patient complain of?

3 What is Leriche's syndrome?

## Answers page 1

**A**

1  Fluid thrill.

2  This patient may also have abdominal distension, dullness in the flanks and shifting dullness.

3  The causes of ascites:
   - infection – tuberculous peritonitis
   - congestive – right-sided heart failure, constrictive pericarditis, Budd–Chiari syndrome
   - hepatic – cirrhosis with portal hypertension, hypoalbuminaemia (from any cause)
   - others – chylous ascites (lymphatic obstruction or transection), Meig's syndrome, pseudomyxoma peritonei, pancreatic disease, intra-abdominal malignancy (especially with peritoneal seedlings).

**B**

1  Left inguinal and right femoral herniae.

2  On examination the inguinal hernia lies above and medial to the pubic tubercle, while the femoral hernia lies below and lateral.

3  Intestinal obstruction and strangulation, the femoral hernia being at particular risk.

**C**

1  There are several stenotic lesions of the right superficial femoral artery.

2  Mild ischaemia causes intermittent claudication, usually in the calf, though the thigh and buttocks may also be involved. More severe symptoms include rest pain in the affected limb, skin changes (thin atrophic skin which is easily damaged, cracks in the heel, brittle deformed nails and ulceration) and gangrene.

3  This is impotence associated with atheromatous occlusion of the abdominal aorta.

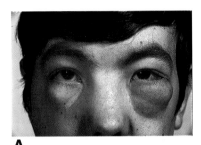

**A**

1   What is the diagnosis?
2   What are the clinical features?

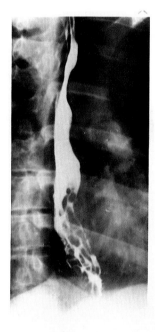

**B**

1   What is this investigation called?
2   What does it show?
3   What are the risk factors for developing this condition?

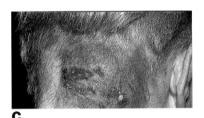

**C**

1   Describe this lesion.
2   What is it called?
3   What is the most likely causative organism?

# Answers page 3

## A

1 Hypertelorism, swelling and central facial deformity, probably a destructive granuloma (Stewart's lethal midline granuloma).

2 Slow, progressive destruction of the midface.

## B

1 A barium swallow.

2 Extensive oesophageal varices in the lower third of the oesophagus.

3 Anything which causes portal hypertension, leading to dilatation of portosystemic venous anastomoses. These can be divided into post-sinusoidal obstruction: e.g. cirrhosis, veno-occlusive disease, hepatic vein obstruction, congestive cardiac failure. Pre-sinusoidal obstruction: e.g. schistosomiasis, congenital hepatic fibrosis, portal vein obstruction. Other causes leading to a high flow state: e.g. tropical splenomegaly or Banti's syndrome.

## C

1 Inflammation of the skin and subcutaneous tissue, with multiple sinuses.

2 Carbuncle.

3 Staphylococcal infection.

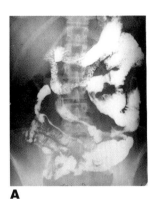

**A**

1 What does this radiograph show?

2 What is the pathology of this disease?

3 What features of this disease may be demonstrable on a radiological contrast study?

4 What is the risk of malignancy with this disease?

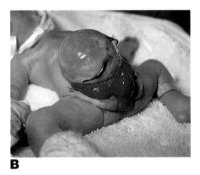

**B**

1 What is the diagnosis?

2 What is its incidence?

3 What are the different types?

4 What other condition is related to this lesion?

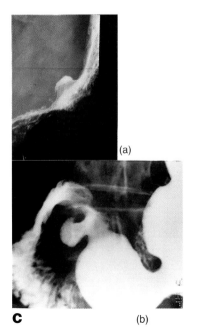

(a)

(b)

**C**

1 What do these radiographs show?

2 What are the different presentations of (a) and (b)?

3 What are the common complications?

# Answers page 5

## A

1  The string sign of Cantor, seen in Crohn's disease of the terminal ileum.

2  Crohn's disease is a chronic granulomatous inflammatory condition that can involve any part of the GI tract from mouth to anus, although commonly it affects the small bowel (hence the term terminal ileitis). The disease occurs in a discontinuous pattern within the bowel and multiple sites are common. Affected areas, however, may be separated by normal bowel (skip lesions). There is transmural chronic inflammation and non-caseating granulomas are pathognomonic, but are absent in up to 40 per cent of specimens.

3  Rose thorn ulcer, fissures, skip lesions, fistulae, thickened mucosa, string sign of Cantor (terminal ileal stricture), featureless drainpipe colon.

4  There is an increased risk of developing carcinoma in colon or small bowel affected by Crohn's disease but the risk of malignancy is less than that of ulcerative colitis.

## B

1  Exomphalos.

2  One in every 6000 births.

3  Exomphalos major is partial or total persistence of midgut within the umbilical cord; exomphalos minor is the herniation of one or two loops of bowel into the base of the cord.

4  Gastroschisis, where loops of bowel herniate through an opening in the abdominal wall: it has no coverings.

## C

1  Peptic ulceration on a barium meal: (a) gastric ulcer, (b) large duodenal ulcer.

2

|  | Gastric | Duodenal |
|---|---|---|
| **Time of pain** | Soon after meals | Two hours after meals |
| **Appetite and weight** | Afraid to eat, with weight loss | Good, with weight gain |
| **Vomiting and haematemesis** | Frequent | Less frequent |

3  Acute: perforation and haemorrhage; chronic: pyloric stenosis, gastric carcinoma and anaemia.

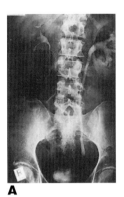

**A**

1  What does this radiograph show?

2  At what three points along the ureter are stones most likely to lodge?

3  What are the other common causes of ureteric obstruction?

4  What are the causes of retroperitoneal fibrosis and what are its complications

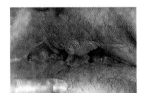

**B**

1  What does this figure show?

2  In what other ways does this disease affect the perianal region?

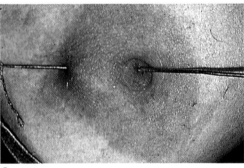

**C**

1  What is this lesion?

2  What is the connecting track?

3  What are the causes of this disease?

# Answers page 7

## A

1  Ureteric stone near the lower end of the left ureter, causing obstruction and dilatation of the ureter and calyces.

2  Stones are most likely to lodge in the pelviureteric junction, where the ureter crosses the sacral promontory and at the vesicoureteric junction.

3  ● Intraluminal – renal and ureteric stones; clot; sloughed renal papilla
   ● intramural – pelviureteric obstruction; ureterocele; TB or schistosomal strictures; surgical damage
   ● extramural - abdominal and pelvic neoplasms and retroperitonal fibrosis.

4  Retroperitoneal fibrosis is a rare condition. In the majority of cases the cause is unknown but in some instances it may be related to an inflammatory abdominal aortic aneurysm, malignant infiltration or the drug methysergide. It leads to bilateral ureteric obstruction, producing a progressive obstructive hydronephrosis and renal failure

## B

1  Perianal Crohn's disease.

2  The spectrum of perianal Crohn's disease may be divided into primary conditions, e.g. fistulae, ulcerated piles, cavitating ulcers; or secondary conditions, e.g. skin tags, strictures, fistulae or abscesses

## C

1  Mammary fistula.

2  The granulomatous track connects a mammary duct and the surface of the breast.

3  Recurrent infection, causing recurrent acute breast abscesses.

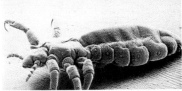

**A**

1   Describe this lesion.

2   What is the most likely diagnosis?

3   How would you treat the condition?

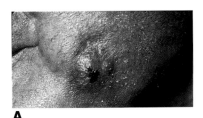

(a)

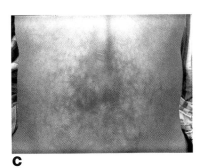

**B**                                    (b)

1   What do figures (a) and (b) show?

2   To what group do these parasites belong?

3   What effects do these parasites produce?

**C**

1   What does this figure of a patient with low back pain show?

2   What is the explanation of pain in his buttocks?

3   What other signs may be present?

# Answers page 9

## A

1  Red induration with a necrotic centre and bloody discharge.

2  Osteomyelitis of the jaw, secondary to a tooth abscess.

3  A chronic abscess and sterile collections resolve only after adequate drainage and debridement. They will not resolve if foreign bodies such as prostheses, mesh, bone sequestra, necrotic tendon or an infected root remain.

## B

1  (a) Head louse;
   (b) head lice in situ.

2  Jointed arthropods.

3  Their bites may be painful and cause hypersensitivity and itching. They may also carry diseases, particularly epidemic typhus and relapsing fever.

## C

1  Erythema ab igne following the application of a hot water bottle to relieve pain in the area.

2  Radiation of pain along the nerve tract, which is compressed.

3  Motor and sensory changes in the limbs.

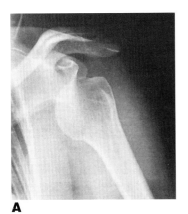

**A**

1   Describe this figure.

2   What are the commonest complications of this condition?

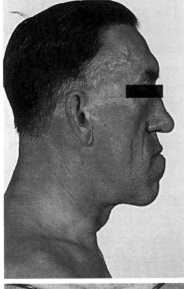

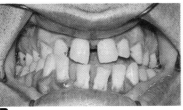

**B**

1   What is this condition?

2   What clinical features are shown in these figures?

3   What neurological problems can this disease cause and why?

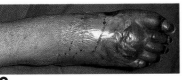

**C**

1   What is the diagnosis?

2   How does this condition develop?

3   What are the clinical signs?

# Answers page 11

### A

1  Dislocation of the left shoulder. Loss of contour of the deltoid muscle owing to displacement of the underlying head of the humerus.

2  ● Axillary nerve palsy
   ● supraspinatus tear
   ● fracture of the surgical neck or greater tuberosity of the humerus.

### B

1  Acromegaly.

2  The features shown include:
   (a) thickened, greasy skin
   (b) prognathism
   (c) an enlarged skull
   (d) prominent lips, nose and tongue.

3  Nerve entrapment problems due to overgrowth of bone and soft tissue. For example, carpal tunnel syndrome, spinal nerve compression giving rise to sciatica, brachial neuropathy and nerve pain and compression of the optic chiasm producing visual disturbances

### C

1  Venous gangrene of the foot.

2  Massive iliofemoral thrombosis or compression from malignancy obstructs venous return, leading to phlegmasia cerulea dolens in extreme cases.

3  The lower limb becomes deeply cyanotic and oedematous. The swollen part is tense, firm and rubbery. Peripheral pulses are lost owing to swelling but the limb remains warm. Shock and toxaemia progress as ischaemia develops and these may lead to venous gangrene.

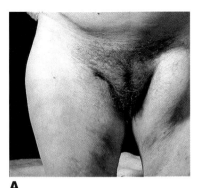

**A**

1 What is this swelling?

2 What are the signs and symptoms of strangulation?

3 Describe the boundaries of this swelling.

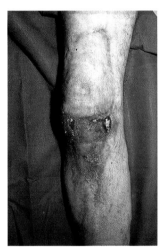

**B**

1 What is the most likely diagnosis in this patient with a six-month history of discharging sinuses?

2 What are the causes of chronic inflammation?

3 What would you expect the cause of this lesion to be?

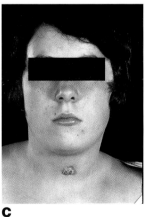

**C**

1 Describe this lesion.

2 What particular care should be taken when removing this lesion?

# Answers page 13

## A

1  Left femoral hernia – the lesion is larger than usual. It also demonstrates how the lesion bulges upwards over the inguinal ligament, making the differential diagnosis with inguinal hernia more difficult. However, an inguinal hernia would have passed more medially into the region of the labia majora.

2  The hernia is irreducible, tense and tender; pain is severe and comes in frequent spasms or can become constant and localized. Signs suggesting involvement of a larger segment of bowel include: elevation of temperature and pulse rate; tenderness, rigidity or rebound tenderness; a raised white cell count; a state of shock; persistent pain for more than two hours after effective gastroduodenal suction has been established.

3  The boundaries of a femoral hernia are ligamentous, except laterally where the boundary is the femoral vein. Medially, lacunar ligament; anteriorly, inguinal ligament; posteriorly pectineal ligament. The ligamentous components make strangulation more likely than with an inguinal hernia.

## B

1  Osteomyelitis of the right tibia with discharging sinuses.

2  Chronic inflammation may be due to failure of an abscess to drain completely, or organisms may be retained in the fibrotic wall of an abscess or within necrotic bone (sequestrum). Such organisms are inaccessible to antibodies and antibiotics owing to the poor blood supply of these areas.

3  Chronic abscesses and sterile collections only resolve after adequate drainage and debridement. This healing does not occur if foreign bodies such as prostheses, mesh, bone sequestra or necrotic tendon remain.

## C

1  Midline cervical cutaneous nodule with scab and scarring, owing to incomplete removal of a thyroglossal cyst.

2  The cyst must be removed completely, following the track to its termination. This may require removal of the central part of the body of the hyoid bone.

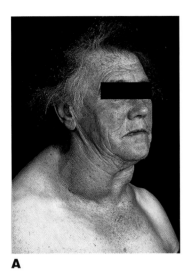

**A**

1   What is the differential diagnosis of this solitary thyroid nodule?

2   What is the significance of a solitary nodule that has been present for seven years without symptoms?

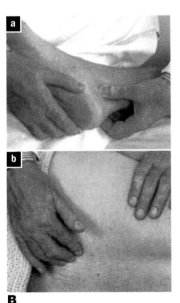

**B**

1   What do these figures show?

2   What is the cause of oedema?

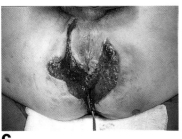

**C**

1   Describe this surgical procedure undertaken for a fistula in ano.

2   How do you explain the size of the wound compared with the size of the lesion?

3   What is meant by Goodsall's rule?

# Answers page 15

## A

1  A solitary nodule may be a non-toxic, benign nodule; toxic; an adenoma; papillary or follicular carcinoma or thyroiditis.

2  About 10 per cent of solitary nodules are carcinomas, the incidence being higher in children and the elderly

## B

1  Digital pressure leaving skin dents around the ankles, on either side of the tendo Achilles and over the sacrum after recumbency.

2  It may result from salt and water retention in cardiac and some renal diseases. Oedema in liver failure relates to low plasma albumin but also interferes with aldosterone metabolism. Oedema accompanies hypoproteinaemia of gut origin, e.g. starvation, malnutrition, malabsorption and protein-losing enteropathies. It accumulates around the feet and ankles of an ambulant patient, over the sacrum in bedridden patients and, in severe cases, in pulmonary oedema.

## C

1  Surgical laying open of a horseshoe-shaped anal fistula, with a posterior midline communication.

2  The extent of the various extensions.

3  For openings anterior to a transverse mid-anal line, the fistula usually runs radially into the anal canal; for openings posterior to this imaginary line, the track is usually curvilinear to open into the anal lumen in the posterior midline. The exceptions to this rule include anterior openings more than 3 cm from the anal margin, which may be anterior extensions of posterior horseshoe fistulae, fistulae associated with Crohn's disease and those arising from carcinoma of the anal glands.

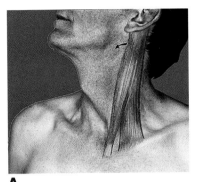

**A**

1  Describe the anatomical regions of the neck.

2  Which triangle of the neck contains the submandibular gland

3  Which triangle of the neck contains a carotid body tumour?

**B**

1  What does this figure show?

2  List the classifications of such a fracture.

3  What are the clinical manifestations?

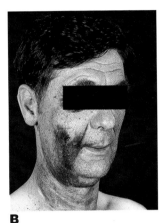

**C**

1  What is the most likely diagnosis of this midline lesion with a cough impulse?

2  Which types of wounds are most prone to this problem?

3  What are the predisposing factors?

# Answers page 17

## A

1  Each side of the neck is divided by the sternomastoid muscle into anterior and posterior triangles. The anterior is also bounded by the midline and the ramus of the mandible and the posterior by the trapezius and the clavicle. The anterior has three subdivisions: the digastric triangle above the two heads of the digastric muscle; the omohyoid, passing downward from the digastric common tendon, divides the remainder of the anterior triangle into a medial muscular triangle and a lateral carotid triangle.

2  The digastric triangle.

3  The carotid triangle.

## B

1  Facial and orbital bruising, oedema and swelling of the cheek, fracture of the right side of the maxilla.

2  Fractures of the maxilla are described according to Le Fort lines, which define the level above which the midfacial skeleton is intact.
   - Line I runs transversely, just above the floor of the nose, through the lower third of the nasal septum
   - line II runs through the bridge of the nose and medial orbital walls via the lachrymal bones
   - line III runs parallel to the base of the skull. The fracture line runs through the nasal bone and continues posteriorly through the ethmoid, crosses the lesser wing of the sphenoid and then runs laterally upwards to the frontozygomatic suture.

3  Unilateral or bilateral periorbital bruising, or unilateral or bilateral gross facial oedema and lengthening of the middle third of the face. Instability of the central bones can interfere with the airway.

## C

1  Abdominal incisional hernia.

2  Vertical rather than transverse wounds.

3  (a) The wound closure technique, i.e. method of closure and drainage
   (b) the general condition of the patient: obesity, jaundice, anaemia, coughing, straining, abdominal distension, vomiting and wound infection.

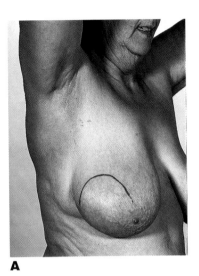

**A**

1   What does this figure show?

2   In which position would abnormalities in a large, pendulous breast become more evident?

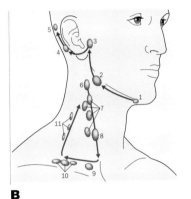

**B**

1   What does this diagram show?

2   What are the common causes of lymphadenopathy?

3   To what do the numbers 6 and 8 refer?

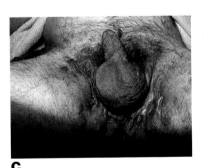

**C**

1   What is the most likely diagnosis?

2   Which part of the skin is affected?

3   Which age group is most commonly affected?

4   What are the predisposing factors?

# Answers page 19

## A

1   Carcinoma of the right breast. On elevation of the arm, cutaneous and deep fixity can be observed.

2   Abnormalities are more evident if the patient leans forward so that the breasts fall away from the body

## B

1   Distribution of lymph nodes in the neck.

2   ● Acute inflammation associated with infection of the ears, nose, throat and skin and subcutaneous tissues
   ● chronic inflammation resulting from TB and sarcoidosis
   ● Hodgkin's and non-Hodgkin's lymphomas
   ● metastatic disease from carcinoma of the upper aerodigestive tract, skin and subcutaneous tumours of the head and neck, and occasionally from other sites, such as breast and upper abdomen.

3   6 – Jugulodigastric node;
   8 – Jugulo-omohyoid node.

## C

1   Hydradenitis suppurativa.

2   It is a chronic suppurative disease of apocrine gland-bearing skin – apocrinitis.

3   Hydradenitis is not seen before puberty and most patients are aged 16–40.

4   Obesity, acne, poor hygiene and excessive sweating have been suggested as predisposing factors.

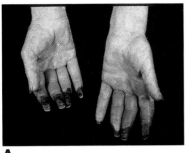

**A**

1   What is the diagnosis?
2   What may cause this condition?

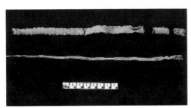

**B**

1   What is the name of this worm?
2   What is the most likely secondary host?
3   What are the symptoms produced by this worm?

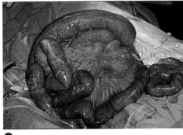

**C**

1   What are the causes of acute intestinal ischaemia?
2   What is the differential diagnosis of acute large bowel ischaemia?
3   What is the typical presentation of a patient with acute ischaemic small bowel?

# Answers page 21

## A

1  Gangrene of the fingertips.

2  Collagen diseases, e.g. rheumatoid arthritis or scleroderma, malignancy, proximal arterial diseases, e.g. embolism, thoracic outlet syndrome, compartment syndrome.

## B

1  *Taenia saginatum*

2  Cattle are the secondary host and the adult tapeworm is found in the human alimentary tract.

3  The symptoms are usually mild, although sometimes a severe anaemia occurs.

## C

1  These can be divided into occlusive, e.g. embolism or thrombosis, and non-occlusive causes, e.g. gut spasm secondary to bacterial toxins or ergot poisoning. The small bowel can also be affected by adhesions or bands, hernias which become strangulated, vasculitis, drugs, trauma, radiotherapy and haemodynamic abnormalities.

2  Late onset ulcerative colitis, Crohn's disease or malignancy.

3  A patient may complain of sudden onset of pain, diarrhoea and vomiting. The patient is unwell, with an increased heart rate, low blood pressure, but initially the abdomen is non-tender. Fever is usually a late development, as peritonitis occurs. There is a high mortality associated with this condition.

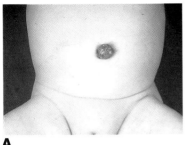

**A**

1 What is the diagnosis of this lesion, which was accompanied by a urinary leak?
2 What is the related internal organ?
3 What would you expect the state of the surrounding skin to be?

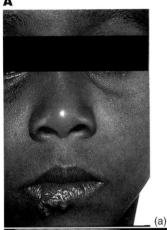

(a)

**B** (b)

1 What is the diagnosis of lesions (a) and (b)?
2 What is the causative micro-organism?

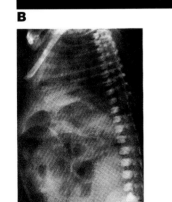

**C**

1 What is the likely diagnosis in this three-day-old infant with abdominal distension and a history of failure to pass meconium rectally?
2 What are the causes of neonatal intestinal obstruction?

# Answers page 23

## A

1  Umbilical polyp associated with urachal fistula.

2  Urinary bladder by way of the urachus.

3  Infective dermatitis is usually associated with this condition.

## B

1  Rounded, elevated ulcer and papillomatous lesions of the lip and of the limb, caused by yaws.

2  *Treponema pertenue.*

## C

1  Meconium ileus.

2  Duodenal atresia, duodenal bands, annular pancreas, Ladd's band, midgut volvulus, meconium ileus secondary to cystic fibrosis, strangulated hernia.

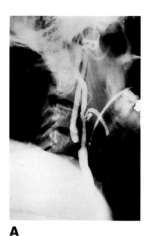

**A**

1  What does this arteriogram show?
2  How may this lesion affect the patient?
3  What other investigations aid the diagnosis of this condition?

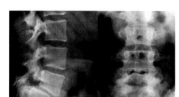

**B**

1  What do these radiographs show?
2  What is the diagnosis?
3  How is this disorder classified?
4  How does it present?

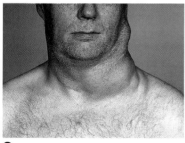

**C**

1  Excisional biopsy of this lesion revealed a low grade lymphoma: how is this disease classified?
2  What is the differential diagnosis?

# Answers page 25

## A

1  A tight stenosis at the origin of the internal carotid artery.

2  These are often asymptomatic. Patients may have transient ischaemic attacks, causing contralateral sensory or motor disturbances, ipsilateral visual loss (amaurosis fugax), speech problems and non-focal symptoms such as memory loss, dizziness and headache. The patient may have an irreversible stroke.

3  Doppler flow studies and CT scan to delineate any damage to the CNS.

## B

1  The forward slippage of one vertebra on another.

2  Spondylolisthesis.

3  The five major types are: congenital, isthmic, traumatic, degenerative and pathological.

4  Patients present with back pain. Examination reveals localized lumbar pain, paraspinal muscle spasm and there may be decreased forward flexion of the spine. Radiologically, oblique radiographs confirm the pars defect as a fracture in the neck of the 'Scottie dog'.

## C

1  Hodgkin's lymphoma - characterized by the binucleate Reed–Sternberg cell, which does not carry B- or T-cell identity.
   Non-Hodgkin's lymphoma
      low grade:  lymphocytic
                  immunocytic (Waldenström's macroglobulinaemia, myeloma)
                  follicular
                  high grade:  centroblastic
                  immunoblastic
                  adult T-cell leukaemia / lymphoma syndrome
                  Burkitt's lymphoma.

2  Lymphadenopathy, carotid body tumour, aneurysm, branchial cyst.

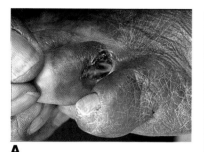

**A**

1   What does this figure show?

2   What are the characteristic features of this type of ulcer?

3   What is the pathophysiology behind the formation of such ulcers and what is the preferred treatment?

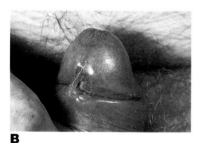

**B**

1   Bacterial examination of this lesion revealed *Haemophilus ducreyi* - what is this ulcer called?

2   Describe the lesion.

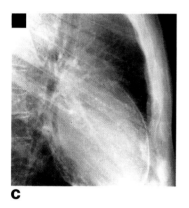

**C**

1   Describe the cardiac abnormality in this radiograph.

2   What are the likely associated clinical signs?

3   What ECG changes would you expect to find?

# Answers page 27

## A

1  An ischaemic ulcer on the fourth toe.

2  This is a full thickness, punched-out lesion with exposure of tendons, ligaments, joints and bone.

3  An inadequate blood supply to the area leads to failure of healing, limited bleeding and lack of a purulent response. Revascularization of the limb will lead to demarcation of viable and non-viable tissue. Healing of the ulcer may then occur. If not, the affected part may have to be amputated.

## B

1  Chancroid.

2  Chancroid is a painful lesion, softer and less indurated than a primary syphilitic lesion. The chancre may be multiple and regional lymph nodes involved may suppurate.

## C

1  Calcification around the myocardium, most probably a calcified pericardium.

2  Calcification and fibrosis (constriction pericarditis) interferes particularly with right ventricular contraction, producing heart failure, with a raised JVP, a large liver, jaundice, ascites and peripheral oedema.

3  Reduced voltage, ST elevation and changes in the T-wave.

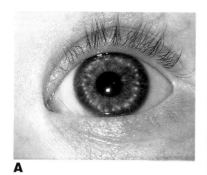

**A**

1  What is the name given to this clinical finding?

2  What chromosomal abnormality is associated with this finding?

3  What other eye signs are associated with this syndrome?

4  What cardiac anomalies are found in this syndrome?

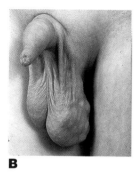

**B**

1  What is the diagnosis?

2  Why do these lesions mainly occur on the left?

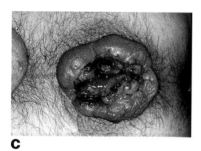

**C**

1  What is the most likely diagnosis?

2  How does this patient present?

3  How would you manage this case?

# Answers page 29

## A

1  Brushfield spots.

2  Trisomy 21, i.e. Down's syndrome.

3  Hypertelorism, prominent epicanthic folds, squint, nystagmus, myopia, keratoconus in adults.

4  Cardiac anomalies are present in 40 per cent of individuals with Down's syndrome. The most commonly found are atrial and ventricular septal defects. Rarer anomalies include a persistent ductus ateriosus and Fallot's tetralogy.

## B

1  Left varicocele.

2  Because the left testicular vein enters the left renal vein and there is often incompetence of venous valves at that junction. The left testicular vein enters the left renal vein at a more vertical angle than the right testicular entering the IVC. The left renal vein is crossed and may be compressed by the pelvic colon and the left testicular vein is longer than the right.

## C

1  Strangulated haemorrhoids.

2  The patient usually presents at the Accident and Emergency department complaining of severe, constant, unremitting pain, a large pile mass protruding from the anal orifice, with gross oedema and, later, ulceration.

3  Controlling pain and discomfort with analgesia and local ice packs; surgical treatment of the piles.

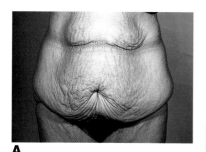

**A**

1  What does this figure show?
2  What significant problems could lie behind it?

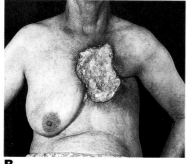

**B**

1  What does this figure show?
2  Which stage of the disease produces this change?

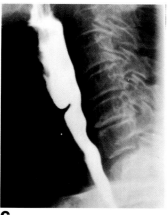

**C**

1  What is this lesion?
2  In which syndrome does it occur?
3  What are the features of the lesion?

# Answers page 31

## A

1  A fatty apron.

2  A fatty apron may cover unsuspected groin pathology, e.g. a femoral hernia.

## B

1  Extensive, neglected malignant ulcer replacing the left breast.

2  A late stage of the disease (stage III;T4), where the underlying neoplasm gives rise to necrosis of the overlying skin and fixity to underlying muscles.

## C

1  This is a post-cricoid oesophageal web.

2  Plummer–Vinson syndrome (sideropenic dysphagia, or Paterson–Kelly syndrome).

3  The patient is usually a middle-aged woman complaining of choking and delayed swallowing at the level of the cricoid cartilage. There is also angular stomatitis, koilonychia, achlorhydria, glossitis and iron deficiency anaemia. This is an important condition because it is pre-malignant and one of the risk factors for developing oesophageal carcinoma.

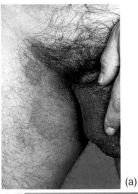

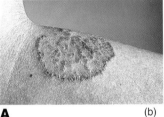

(a)

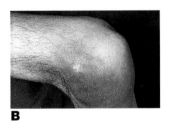

**A**            (b)

1. What are the most likely diagnoses in figures (a) and (b)?
2. What is the causative agent?

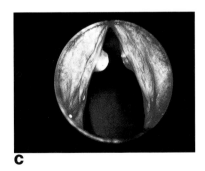

**B**

1. What is the most likely diagnosis in this patient with known pulmonary tuberculosis?
2. What is meant by a chronic abscess?
3. What are the causes of the chronic inflammatory process?

**C**

1. What does this figure show?
2. What predisposes to this condition?
3. How may this condition present clinically

# Answers page 33

## A

1 (a) Tinea cruris;
  (b) Tinea corporis.

2 Both are cutaneous fungal infections (mycosis).

## B

1 Tuberculosis of the tibia.

2 When an inflammatory process lasts for a number of weeks or longer it is termed chronic.

3 Chronic inflammation is seen in:
  - the presence of endogenous or exogenous substances, such as hair, keratin, uric acid crystals, suture material, prostheses, asbestos and silica
  - certain organisms, e.g. tuberculosis, syphilis, fungi and parasites
  - autoimmune disease, e.g. rheumatoid arthritis, chronic hepatitis and thyroiditis
  - some diseases of unknown aetiology, e.g. Crohn's, sarcoid and Wegener's granulomatosis.

## C

1 Singer's nodes.

2 Excessive use and straining of the voice. (This disease is therefore very common in singers, actors and teachers.)

3 It commonly presents as hoarseness, either acutely after an episode of vocal straining or insidiously over weeks or months.

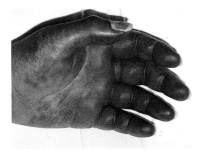

**A**

1 What is this condition and what is its aetiology?
2 In whom does it occur?
3 What is the management?

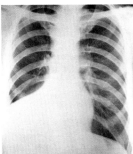

**B**

1 These are chest X-rays of patients with atelectasis. What is this condition?
2 What are the common causes?
3 What is the treatment?

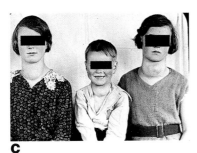

**C**

1 What does this figure show?
2 What is the pathology of this condition?
3 How do these patients present?

# Answers page 35

## A

1  Venous gangrene of the hand secondary to axillary vein thrombosis.

2  Patients who have done some unusual or excessive exercise, often involving holding the arm above the head, e.g. painters or decorators. Most commonly it affects men aged 35–45 years. The first recorded case was in King Henry II of France, who developed the condition through waving his sword above his head! It may also occur in patients with cervical ribs or thoracic inlet obstruction and by external compression of the vein, e.g. Pancoast tumour of the lung or enlarged malignant axillary lymph nodes.

3  Early or acute management involves brachial venography, followed by thrombolysis (streptokinase or urokinase), followed by several months of anticoagulation. Decompression of the thoracic inlet may be indicated. Most patients become symptom-free after a few months owing to the development of collateral venous drainage. If discomfort and oedema persist, it is possible to bypass the obstruction.

## B

1  A collapse of all or part of a lung, following occlusion to part of the bronchial tree.

2  Perioperatively it may occur during anaesthesia. Most commonly it occurs postoperatively, secondary to poor expansion of the lungs because of pain, which causes mucous plug retention within the bronchial tree and therefore occlusion. It may also be caused by inhalation of a foreign body or secondary to a bronchial neoplasm.

3  Postoperative causes can be treated with chest physiotherapy, deep breathing, analgesia and mucous plug extraction by bronchoscopy if needed. A foreign body is treated by bronchoscopic extraction.

## C

1  Multinodular goitre in siblings with deficiency goitres.

2  Multinodular goitre results from disordered thyroid metabolism, where some areas of the gland become hyperplastic and form nodules which later degenerate, fibrose or calcify. Multinodular goitre may arise primarily or develop from a pre-existing smooth enlargement.

3  The swelling may be asymptomatic or produce dysphagia, dyspnoea or stridor from tracheal compression. Secondary thyrotoxicosis may develop in a pre-existing multinodular goitre, causing symptoms of weight loss, diarrhoea, heat intolerance, sweating, tremor, weakness, palpitations, arrhythmias and ophthalmic signs.

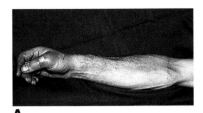

**A**

1  What does the figure show?

2  What should you include in your examination?

3  What are the signs?

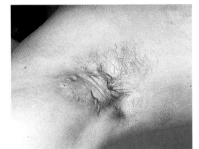

**B**

1  What is the most likely diagnosis?

2  What sites are usually involved?

3  What is the aetiology of such a lesion?

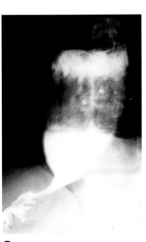

**C**

1  What does this barium swallow show?

2  What is the pathophysiology of this condition?

3  What is Chagas' disease?

# Answers page 37

## A

1 Swollen, infected right thumb with tell-tale red lines due to lymphangitis.

2 Apart from the local examination, the possibility of regional node enlargement should be suspected and examined for.

3 Locally: redness, swelling, tenderness and pain; systemically: pyrexia, malaise.

## B

1 Suppurative hydradenitis of the right axilla.

2 The axilla is the most common site but the groin, umbilicus, back of the neck and the perineum may be affected.

3 Bacterial infection of a plugged apocrine gland, then abscess formation with subsequent drainage and sinus formation. Repeated infection creates a wide area of inflamed and scarred tissue which is foul smelling and painful.

## C

1 There is gross dilatation of the oesophagus, with smooth tapering to a stenosis. This is typical of achalasia.

2 There is an aganglionic defect in Auerbach's plexus of vagal fibres around the oesophagus: this is thought to be viral in origin and causes disordered oesophageal motility. Initially there are simultaneous non-peristaltic contractions of the oesophagus, the oesophagus then dilates, accompanied by dysphagia and regurgitation of food. Monometry shows a high resting oesophageal pressure with absent peristalsis.

3 This is an infection by *Trepanosoma cruzi*, which is common in South America. Ganglion cells are destroyed, causing features of achalasia and megaoesophagus. It can also produce megaduodenum, megacolon and megaureter.

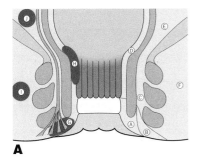

**A**

1  What does this figure show?

2  What are G, H, I and J?

3  What are the spaces A, B, C, D, E and F?

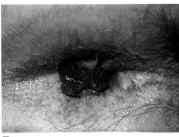

**B**

1  What is the most likely diagnosis?

2  What are the manifestations of the disease?

3  How would you treat this patient?

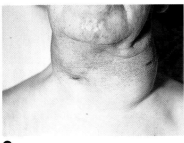

**C**

1  What is the most probable diagnosis of this fixed, stony hard neck mass?

2  How does it spread?

3  Which age group is most commonly affected?

# Answers page 39

**A**

1  Anatomy of the anal region.

2  G – perianal; H – submucosal; I – ischiorectal; J – pelvirectal abscesses.

3  A – marginal; B – perianal; C – intersphincteric; D – submucosal;
   E – supralevator (pararectal); F – ischiorectal fossa.

**B**

1  Third degree haemorrhoids.

2  Rectal bleeding; an irreducible anal lump.

3  Surgical intervention is the best option for third degree haemorrhoids.

**C**

1  Anaplastic carcinoma of the thyroid.

2  It spreads rapidly: most patients with anaplastic carcinoma die within
   one year. Locally it invades the trachea and oesophagus.

3  It appears between the ages of 60 and 80.

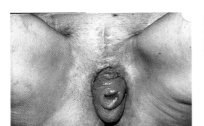

**A**

1 What is this vaginal protrusion?
2 What are the predisposing factors?

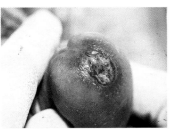

(a)

(b)

**B**

1 What is the most likely common diagnosis in these figures?
2 What is the organism involved?
3 Describe the lesion of the penis?

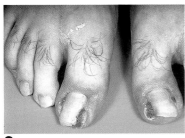

**C**

1 What is the diagnosis?
2 What are the predisposing factors?

# Answers page 41

## A

1  Vaginal procidentia.

2  When the pelvic diaphragm and the ligaments supporting the uterus are defective the cervix appears at the introitus on straining and becomes extruded to a varying degree.

## B

1  Primary syphilitic infection of the penis and primary chancre of the lower lip.

2  The spirochaete *Treponema pallidum.*

3  An ulcerated lesion with a sloping edge and blood-stained discharge, accompanied by regional lymphadenopathy. The inguinal nodes affected become hard and shotty.

## C

1  Ingrowing toenail.

2  Excessive outgrowth of the nail into the nail fold, precipitated by tight shoes, or cutting the corner of the toenail. The sharp edge then penetrates the nail fold, as it grows forward rather than growing clear of the skin.

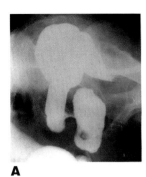

**A**

1   What is the abnormality shown in this radiograph?

2   What may predispose to this condition?

3   What is the treatment?

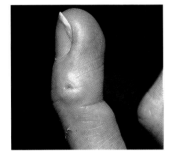

**B**

A nurse working with many infected wounds developed this hand infection.

1   Describe the lesion.

2   What is the diagnosis?

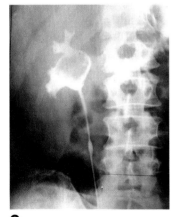

**C**

1   What does this IVU show?

2   What is the most likely diagnosis?

3   What is the treatment?

# Answers page 43

## A

1  A vesicocolic fistula.

2  Colonic causes include diverticulitis, carcinoma of the colon or rectum and Crohn's disease. Other causes include transitional cell carcinoma of the bladder, trauma and post-radiotherapy.

3  These lesions do not close spontaneously so surgery is the main option. The colonic lesion is resected, with defunctioning colostomy, and the bladder is closed with omental interposition and catheter drainage.

## B

1  A whitish punctated lesion of the digit.

2  Herpetic whitlow. The initial blister usually becomes secondarily infected and takes a number of weeks to heal.

## C

1  There is a filling defect in the right renal pelvis.

2  Transitional cell carcinoma of the renal pelvis.

3  A nephroureterectomy.

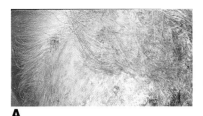

**A**

1 What is the most likely diagnosis in this patient with known syphilis?

2 What are the stages of the disease?

3 What other sites are likely to be involved at this stage of the disease?

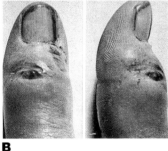

**B**

1 What is the diagnosis?

2 What is the difference between this lesion and a terminal pulp space infection?

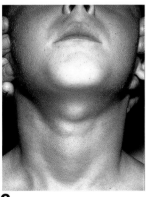

**C**

1 What is the diagnosis?

2 How can you confirm this clinically?

3 What is the embryology of this condition?

# Answers page 45

## A

1  Gummatous syphilitic lesion of the scalp.

2  Primary lesion: one week to three months after inoculation; secondary: generalized disease accompanied by fever, malaise, skin rash and general lymphadenopathy; tertiary: gummatous stage – the classical tertiary lesions are found in the skull.

3  Cardiovascular system: involving the ascending aorta and may produce a superior mediastinal aneurysm; central nervous system: neurosyphilis comprising general paralysis of the insane, tabes dorsalis and meningovascular disease.

## B

1  Infection over the proximal phalanx.

2  Both have a similar aetiology and clinical course, but in this infection oedema is more marked because of skin laxity.

## C

1  Suprahyoid thyroglossal cyst.

2  The cyst moves upward on swallowing and on protrusion of the tongue.

3  The thyroid develops from a cell mass arising at the base of the tongue and descends to its anatomical position anterior to the third and fourth tracheal rings along the thyroglossal tract. Normally the tract should atrophy completely. Failure to do this results in a thyroglossal cyst. Ninety per cent are found in front of the hyoid bone, 8 per cent below it and 2 per cent lingually.

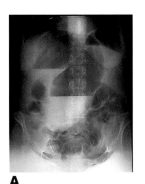

**A**

1 What does this radiograph show?
2 How may this condition occur?
3 How may this patient present?

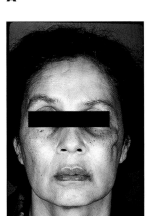

**B**

1 What is this injury?
2 How do these injuries present?
3 What are the differential diagnoses?

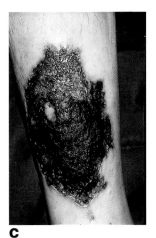

**C**

1 What is the most likely diagnosis?
2 What is the predisposing factor for its development?
3 What is the difference between this lesion and synergistic gangrene?

# Answers page 47

## A

1  Caecal volvulus.

2  This occurs in those whose right colon has a mesentery continuous with that of the small bowel. Also the caecum does not occupy its normal position in the right iliac fossa.

3  The patient may present with signs of large bowel obstruction (i.e. abdominal pain, distension, absolute constipation and vomiting). On examination there is usually a distended, tense, palpable resonant mass filling the centre of the abdomen, with an empty, concave right iliac fossa.

## B

1  Fracture of the left zygoma.

2  A zygomatic fracture presents alone, or associated with a Le Fort fracture. It presents with facial oedema, periorbital bruising at the site of the injury and may involve the temporomandibular joint, with painful mastication, numbness of the cheek because of damage to the infraorbital nerve and diplopia from displacement of the lateral suspensory ligament of the eyeball.

3  Fracture of the left maxilla, or a combination of fractures of the maxilla and zygoma.

## C

1  Pyoderma gangrenosum.

2  Depression of the immune system; associated diseases include Crohn's disease, ulcerative colitis, rheumatoid arthritis, plasma cell dyscrasia and leukaemia.

3  Pyoderma gangrenosum has a similar acute pathology to synergistic gangrene which is related to recent wounds.

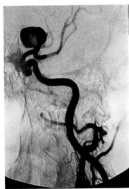

**A**

1   What is this investigation and what does it show?

2   How may this condition present?

3   What conditions are associated with aneurysms?

**B**

1   What does this figure show?

2   What are the predisposing factors for this disease?

3   What is the distribution of this disease within the large bowel?

4   What are the five-year survival rates for this disease in relation to Duke's classification?

**C**

1   This is a Volkmann's contracture of the upper limb. What is the pathophysiology?

2   What are the causes of Volkmann's ischaemic contracture?

3   What is the treatment?

# Answers page 49

## A

1   It is an arteriogram showing a berry aneurysm.

2   Cerebrovascular accident, subarachnoid haemorrhage, effects caused by pressure on surrounding brain tissue or an incidental finding on a CT scan.

3   Atherosclerosis and all its predisposing factors, e.g. male sex, smoking, diabetes, hypercholesterolaemia, hypertension, genetic predisposition, connective tissue diseases, e.g. Ehlers–Danlos syndrome, Marfan's syndrome, pseudoxanthoma elasticum, syphilis, congenital or berry aneurysm.

## B

1   Colonic neoplasm seen at time of colonoscopy.

2   (a)Environmental factors include a lack of fibre, thus increasing transit time and allowing increased exposure of gut mucosa to carcinogens and also bile acids. Bile acids have both an indirect effect of bacteria converting the bile acids to carcinogens and also a direct toxic effect on the mucosa.
    (b)Inflammatory bowel disease: ulcerative colitis. (The relationship between colonic carcinoma and Crohn's disease is still controversial.)
    (c)Irradiation: there is an increased incidence in patients who have undergone previous pelvic irradiation.
    (d)Genetic factors: familial adenomatous polyposis (an autosomal dominant condition - location on chromosome 5). A group of patients with non-hereditary polyposis coli also have a predisposition to large bowel tumours. There is greater incidence in people who have siblings or first degree relatives with colonic carcinoma.

3   Approximately 45 per cent of tumours are situated in the rectum. Within the colon: 25 per cent occur in the sigmoid colon, 15 per cent in the caecum or ascending colon and 10 per cent in the transverse colon. The remaining 5 per cent are found in the descending colon.

4
| Duke's stage | Definition | Percentage 5-year survival rates |
| --- | --- | --- |
| A | Confined to bowel wall with no involvement of lymph nodes | 90 |
| B | Extension through the wall of the bowel but no involvement of lymph nodes | 70 |
| C1 | Nodes involved locally around the primary growth | 40 |
| C2 | Continuous string of involved nodes up to the proximal limit of resection | 26 |
| D | Distant metastases | 16 |

## C

1   Compression of the muscles within a rigid muscular compartment causes vascular compression and ischaemia with subsequent fibrosis of the muscle. Up to six hours from the event the ischaemia is usually reversible, between six and twelve hours, mottling occurs and the skin becomes firm secondary to oedema. After twelve hours, ischaemic changes become irreversible. Fibrosis and contracture are late sequelae of the syndrome.

2   Embolus, trauma, e.g. major arterial injury, arterial ligation, thrombosis secondary to intimal damage, displaced fracture or dislocation of a joint, tight bandaging or splinting of a fractured limb.

3   Firstly treat the cause. If there is a traumatic element, a fasciotomy is necessary. Once Volkmann's contracture has occurred, the muscle damage is irreversible, but releasing procedures may improve function.

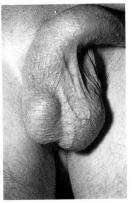

**A**

1  What does the blue line on the skin indicate?

2  What is the differential diagnosis?

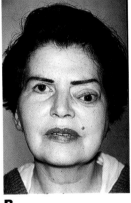

**B**

1  What does this figure show?

2  What types of cysts most commonly occur in the oral/facial region?

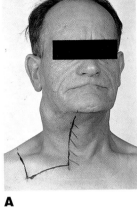

**C**

1  This is a teratoma of the left testis. How may it present?

2  What tumour markers may be positive?

3  How would you manage this disease?

# Answers page 51

## A

1  Tattoo markings for radiotherapy.

2  Primary or secondary malignant lymph nodes.

## B

1  Mucocele in the left frontal sinus bulging into the orbit.

2  Cysts associated with fusion of embryological elements forming the maxilla; cysts of dental origin, which tend to present in the oral cavity; mucocele of paranasal air sinuses resulting from obstruction of the sinus by a polyp and atresia or mucus of the sinus osteum.

## C

1  Ninety per cent of cases occur as a painless enlargement of the testis, which may be accompanied by a heavy or dragging sensation. Ten per cent present as an acutely painful testicle. Many also have an associated hydrocele.

2  Alpha-fetoprotein, non-placental beta-human gonadotrophin, placental alkaline phosphatase and carcinoembryonic antigen.

3  Radical orchidectomy through an inguinal incision, followed by chest X-ray and CT scan of the abdomen and chest to look for hepatic and pulmonary metastases and para-aortic lymph node involvement. This is followed by chemotherapy, usually with cisplatin. Patients are followed up with serial tumour markers to detect recurrence.

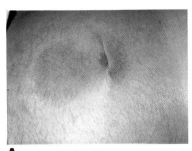

**A**

1 What does this figure show and with what disease is it associated?

2 What criteria are used to determine the severity of this disease?

3 What other abdominal conditions produce a raised serum amylase?

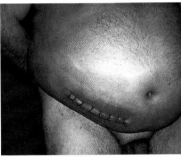

**B**

1 Describe this figure.

2 How is the causative organism classified?

3 What is an abscess?

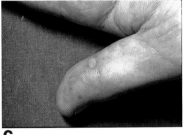

**C**

1 What is the diagnosis of this lesion in a patient with subacute bacterial endocarditis?

2 What other symptoms may be present?

# Answers page 53

## A

1  Cullen's sign, periumbilical staining associated with acute pancreatitis.

2  A number of scoring systems using multiple laboratory criteria have been proposed, of which Imrie's is widely accepted:

- age greater than 55 years
- white blood count greater than $15 \times 10^9 \, l^{-1}$
- glucose greater than 10 mmol $l^{-1}$
- albumin less than 32 g $l^{-1}$
- urea greater than 16 mmol $l^{-1}$
- $Po_2$ less than 8 kPa
- LDH greater than 600 units $l^{-1}$
- AST greater than 200 units $l^{-1}$

The presence of three or more of the above criteria within the first forty-eight hours indicates a severe attack.

3  Perforated peptic ulcer, gall bladder perforation, outlet obstruction following gastrectomy, ruptured abdominal aortic aneurysm, mesenteric infarction, ruptured ectopic pregnancy.

## B

1  An appendix wound, erythema, redness and surrounding swelling, mostly resulting from infection.

2  Commensal. Infection from within the body is called endogenous and from elsewhere exogenous. The commensals are normally resident on the skin in the axillae, in the mucosa of the throat and nose, in the perineum, and in the intestine. Commensals have the potential to become harmful pathogens if they breach the body surface and multiply.

3  An abscess is a collection of unresolved and subcutaneous dead tissue, organisms and other foreign materials.

## C

1  Dissemination of septic emboli may produce deep or superficial lesions.

2  Fever, general malaise and symptoms of cardiac disease.

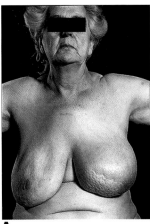

**A**

1 Describe the abnormalities in this figure.

2 What is the most probable diagnosis?

3 What are the factors affecting prognosis?

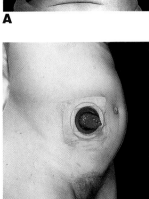

**B**

1 What type of stoma is this?

2 What other types of stoma do you know?

3 Why are ileostomies fashioned with a spout?

4 What are the potential complications of a stoma?

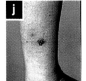

**C**

1 What is this lesion?

2 What features make you suspicious that a naevus is malignant?

3 What is the significance of the thickness of the lesion in a malignant melanoma?

# Answers page 55

## A

1  Bilaterally deformed breasts, with evidence of lumps. Redness and oedema of the left breast, with a swelling protruding from the sternal region.

2  Bilateral carcinoma of the breast, with external protrusion from secondary bone deposits.

3  The stage of the tumour, the number of lymph nodes involved and the presence of distant metastases. In this case the disease is stage IV, with distant metastases (bone involvement), carrying a poor prognosis.

## B

1  Ileostomy.

2  Stomas may be temporary or permanent. Temporary stomas are usually to protect a distal anastomosis and may be single- or double-barrelled. Permanent stomas are necessary when there is no distal bowel segment remaining after resection, or if for some reason the bowel cannot be rejoined. Permanent stomas may be ileostomies or colostomies. Ileostomies are usually fashioned in the right lower abdomen, colostomies in the left iliac fossa.

3  The spout ensures that the irritant small bowel contents enter the ileostomy appliance directly rather than flowing onto the skin.

4  Early complications of a stoma include: oedema, haemorrhage, ulceration, dehiscence of the suture line, ischaemic stenosis. Late complications include: protraction, prolapse and parastomal hernias.

## C

1  Malignant melanoma.

2  Change in size or shape, the naevus may become darker, start bleeding or become itchy, with ulceration and enlarged regional lymph nodes.

3  The thickness of the primary lesion is directly related to the clinical outcome. Less than 0.76 mm thickness is a low risk and patients have an 87 per cent ten-year survival rate; 0.76–1.5 mm has a moderate risk; greater than 1.5 mm thickness is a high risk for the patient, and the ten-year survival rate is 10 per cent if the lesion is greater than 4 mm thick. Note: this does not accurately predict the outcome for an individual patient, as a lesion of any thickness may metastasize.

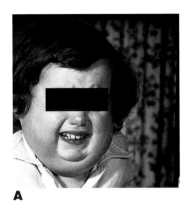

**A**

1 What does this figure show?

2 What organism causes this disease?

3 What other systems can this disease affect?

4 At what age should individuals be vaccinated against this disease? In whom is it contraindicated?

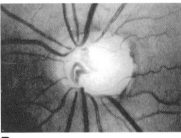

**B**

1 What does this figure show?

2 What is the pathology of this condition?

3 What are the common causes of glaucoma?

4 How may this present clinically?

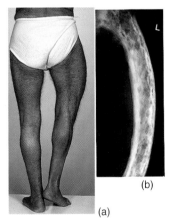

(a)

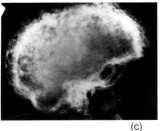

(b)

(c)

1 What is the diagnosis?

2 Describe the radiological changes in (b).

3 What are the complications of this disease?

# Answers page 57

### A

1  Bilateral parotid swellings secondary to mumps.

2  Paramyxovirus.

3  • CNS – meningoencephalitis in 5 per cent of patients
   • GU – epididymo-orchitis in one-third of patients, oophoritis
   • hepatobiliary – hepatitis, pancreatitis
   • CVS – myocarditis
   • musculoskeletal – polyarthritis.

4  Children are vaccinated at the age of twelve to fifteen months with the MMR vaccine and then again with a booster dose at school entry age (three to five years). Contraindications against vaccination include:

   (a) altered immunity or untreated malignant disease
   (b) immunosuppressive treatment, radiotherapy or high-dose corticosteroids
   (c) children who have received another live vaccine within three weeks
   (d) pregnancy.

### B

1  Cupping and optic atrophy in acute glaucoma.

2  A narrow anterior chamber predisposes to acute glaucoma, which results in a rapid rise in intraocular pressure. The loss of vision owing to optic nerve damage may be permanent unless there is prompt intervention and treatment.

3  Glaucoma may be classified as primary or secondary. Primary glaucoma may be congenital, acute (closed angle) or chronic (open angle). Secondary glaucoma may be as a result of iritis, injury, central retinal vein thrombosis or steroid eyedrops.

4  Days or weeks previously, the patient may notice halos (caused by diffraction from an oedematous cornea). There is then rapid loss of vision, accompanied by orbital pain, photophobia and nausea. The eye is red and watery and the pupil may be oval in shape.

### C

1  Paget's disease.

2  The left femur shows thickening, sclerotic changes and bowing.

3  Pathological fracture, spinal stenosis and paraplegia, osteoarthritis, diplopia, deafness and high output cardiac failure; on rare occasions malignant change to an osteosarcoma.

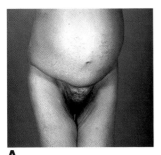

**A**

1   What is this abnormality?

2   What is the differential diagnosis?

3   What signs could be elicited in the patient?

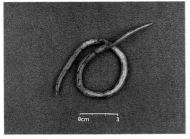

**B**

1   What is this worm?

2   What is its surgical significance?

3   How are worms classified?

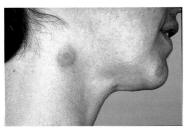

(a)

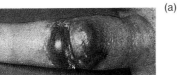

**C**                        (b)

1   What are the common features of figures (a) and (b)?

2   What reactions can be produced by these organisms?

# Answers page 59

## A

1  Ascites. The umbilicus is usually displaced downward by ascites.

2  Ovarian or uterine mass, enlarged bladder, retroperitoneal mass.

3  Shifting dullness and a fluid thrill.

## B

1  *Ascaris lumbricoides* (common roundworm).

2  Large collections lead to internal obstruction. Passing to the lung, they can migrate to the epiglottis. The worm may migrate to the appendix, leading to appendicitis. If it migrates to the pancreatic duct or common bile duct, it may lead to obstructive jaundice.

3  ● Roundworms (nematodes)
   ● tapeworm (cestodes)
   ● flukes (trematodes).

## C

1  Both were produced by insect bites.

2  Reactions to insect bites vary from mild hyperaemia to acute allergic, or local or systemic effects.

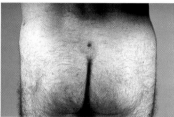

**A**

1  What is the name of the test being performed in this figure?

2  Which part of the leg is being examined?

3  How is the test performed?

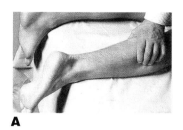

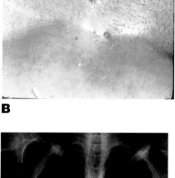

**B**

1  What do these figures show?

2  What is the aetiology of this disease?

3  How do these patients usually present?

4  Where else can this condition occur?

1  Describe this radiograph.

2  What is the causative organism?

3  Which sites are commonly involved?

**C**

# Answers page 61

## A

1  Simmonds' test.

2  The tendo Achillis is being examined for possible rupture.

3  The patient lies prone with the feet hanging over the end of a couch. The calf is squeezed transversely and if the tendon is intact or incompletely ruptured the foot is seen to plantar flex. If the tendon is completely ruptured, there is no movement of the foot.

## B

1  Pilonidal sinus.

2  The aetiology of this disease is unclear. It is suggested that trauma is causative by the fact that the opening is in the natal cleft, at the site of maximal shearing stresses when seated. There is also some debate as to whether the condition is congenital.

3  Patients may be asymptomatic or may present with an acute abscess or a chronic discharging sinus.

4  The condition is also found in hands, the umbilicus and the axillae. It is often seen in the hands of barbers, where hair clippings enter the web of the right hand between the index and ring fingers.

## C

1  A chest radiograph showing a calcified hydatid lung abscess.

2  Larvae of *Echinococcus granulosus* (tapeworm).

3  Liver, lung, kidney and brain are common sites but they may present anywhere in the body.

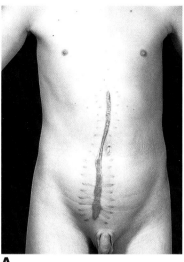

**A**

1  Describe this figure.
2  What are the characteristics of this scar?

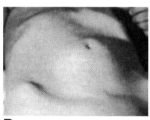

**B**

1  What does this figure of a collapsed 70-year-old man show?
2  What are the differential diagnoses?
3  What is the likely presentation?

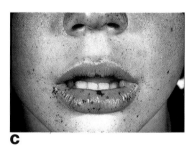

**C**

1  What is the aetiology of this disorder?
2  What is the abnormality shown?
3  What are the associated lesions in the small intestine?
4  List complications of this lesion.

# Answers page 63

### A

1  Right paramedian incision extending from the xiphisternum to the suprapubic region, with a pink hypertrophic scar.

2  This fibrous reaction is limited to the scar, which may be tender and may itch. The scar can continue to enlarge for about six months but regress after a year to pale, thin, stretched scar tissue.

### B

1  The central abdominal mass of a ruptured abdominal aortic aneurysm. The mass is produced by both the aneurysm and the surrounding haematoma.

2  Perforated peptic ulcer, myocardial infarction, pancreatitis, ruptured aortic aneurysm, dissecting aortic aneurysm, spontaneous oesophageal rupture (rare).

3  Acute central abdominal pain radiating through to the back, a state of shock and possibly a prior history of a pulsating abdominal mass.

### C

1  Peutz–Jeghers' syndrome is inherited as autosomal dominant inheritance, with a high degree of penetrance.

2  Perioral pigmentation.

3  Hamartomatous polyposis.

4  (a) Intussusception
   (b) ulceration
   (c) bleeding.

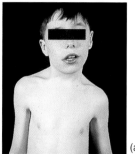
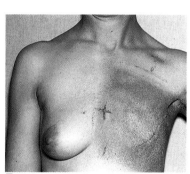

**A**

(a)

(b)

1  What is the common pathology in these two figures?

2  What is the deformity in figures (a) and (b) called?

3  What produces this deformity?

**B**

1  What does this figure show?

2  What skin changes are associated with breast carcinoma?

3  What are the risk factors involved with breast carcinoma?

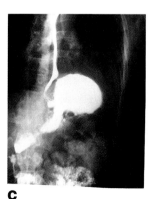

**C**

1  What is the diagnosis?

2  What are the four types of hiatus hernia?

3  Name two operations for this condition.

# Answers page 65

## A

1   Sternomastoid tumour.

2   Torticollis.

3   Torticollis may result from a sternomastoid tumour during childhood and fibrosis or tumours of the sternomastoid in the adult. Lesions adjacent to the muscle may also produce contraction or contractures of the muscle, with resultant deformity.

## B

1   Secondary cutaneous changes following mastectomy and adjuvant radiotherapy to the left breast in the treatment of breast carcinoma.

2   Nipple retraction, peau d'orange, skin tethering or ulceration if the tumour has cutaneous involvement, Paget's disease of the nipple, superficial thrombophlebitis.

3   Hormonal activity or sensitivity, hence associations with female sex, nulliparity, early menarche and late menopause, also links with smoking, obesity, high social class. There is a strong genetic component, with the risk being significantly greater in first degree relatives.

## C

1   Paraoesophageal hiatus hernia.

2   ● Type I or sliding hiatus hernia, which accounts for 85 per cent
    ● type II or rolling (paraoesophageal) hiatus hernia, which accounts for 5 per cent
    ● type III, types I and II occurring together
    ● type IV, where other organs as well as the stomach herniate into the thoracic cavity.

3   Hill gastropexy and Nissen fundoplication. An increasing number of laparascopic fundoplication procedures are being undertaken.

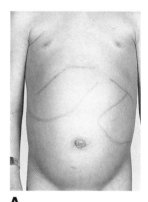

**A**

1 What is the cause of abdominal distension in this patient?

2 What is the classification of this condition?

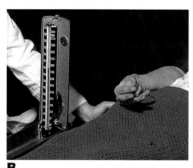

**B**

1 What does this figure show?

2 What other symptoms and signs may be present?

3 What are the common causes?

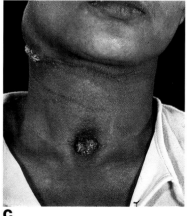

**C**

1 What is meant by scrofula?

2 What is a collar-stud abscess?

3 What is the most likely diagnosis of the lesion shown?

# Answers page 67

## A

1  Hepatosplenomegaly and ascites.
2  Causes of ascites:

| | |
|---|---|
| ● infection | tuberculous peritonitis |
| ● congestive | right-sided heart failure |
| | constrictive pericarditis |
| | Budd–Chiari syndrome |
| ● hepatic | cirrhosis with portal hypertension |
| | hypoalbuminaemia (from any cause) |
| ● others | chylous ascites (lymphatic obstruction or transection) |
| | Meig's syndrome |
| | pseudomyxoma peritonei |
| | pancreatic disease |
| | intra-abdominal malignancy (especially with peritoneal seedlings). |

## B

1  Trousseau's sign – carpal spasm secondary to hypocalcaemia.

2  Chvostek's sign – facial muscle contraction in response to tapping the facial nerve as it emerges in front of the auditory meatus, tetany, orofacial paraesthesia, abdominal cramps.

3  Renal failure, postoperative following parathyroid surgery, acute pancreatitis, pseudohypoparathyroidism (a syndrome of end organ resistance to parathyroid hormone), iatrogenic, e.g. drugs (calcitonin diphosphanates) and citrated blood in massive transfusion.

## C

1  Degenerative lymph nodes.

2  A purulent collection superficial and deep to the deep fascia.

3  Cervical tuberculosis.

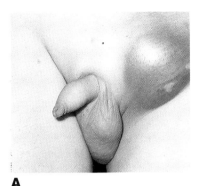

**A**

1  Describe this lesion.

2  What is the most likely diagnosis?

3  Where would you expect the primary lesion to be?

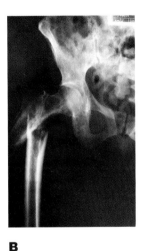

**B**

1  What is the diagnosis?

2  Why has this occurred?

3  Which tumours metastasize commonly to bone?

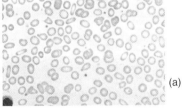

(a)

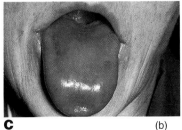

**C**                          (b)

1  How are these figures related?

2  What other conditions can cause this blood picture?

3  How can the causes of this blood picture be distinguished?

# Answers page 69

## A

1  A red, erythematous swelling in the left inguinal region of a young child.

2  Suppurative inguinal nodes.

3  They are mostly secondary to infections in the leg, abdominal wall, penis, scrotum or perineum.

## B

1  Transverse fracture to the upper end of the shaft of the femur (this is a pathological fracture).

2  Metastatic deposits form in the femur, causing weakness to the bone which is easily fractured.

3  Bronchus, thyroid, breast, kidney and prostate. They form lytic lesions in bone, apart from prostate and sometimes breast which form sclerotic lesions. These malignancies commonly metastasize to bones as these organs commonly have a highly developed venous plexus which is in direct communication with the descending venous plexus of the vertebral column.

## C

1  Plummer–Vinson syndrome and microcytic anaemia are both seen in iron deficiency anaemias.

2  Other causes of a microcytic anaemia include thalassaemia, sideroblastic anaemia and anaemia of chronic disease.

3  Measurement of the body iron (including serum iron, total iron binding capacity, serum ferritin and iron stores in the bone marrow) identifies an iron deficiency anaemia. Serum electrophoresis demonstrates haemoglobin abnormalities causing a microcytic picture.

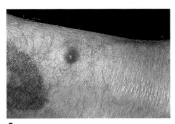

**A**

1 What is this condition?
2 What is a glomus?
3 How do these present clinically?

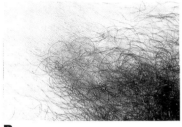

**B**

1 Describe the lesion shown in the figure.
2 What is the most likely diagnosis?
3 What is the probable causative organism?

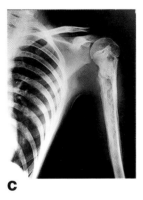

**C**

1 What does this radiograph show?
2 What is the diagnosis?
3 What is the commonest cause of this condition?

# Answers page 71

### A

1  Glomus tumour.

2  A specialized arteriovenous anastomosis found particularly around nail beds and concerned with heat regulation. It is densely innervated.

3  Glomus tumours are subcutaneous, discrete, benign nodules. They can occur anywhere in the body but usually at the extremities of limbs. They are often subungual. The lesions have a bluish tinge because of their blood content and may be extremely sensitive to gentle trauma and temperature change. The patient may complain of a severe or sharp throbbing pain.

### B

1  Red, erythematous induration with a necrotic centre.

2  Inguinal folliculitis.

3  Staphylococcal infection.

### C

1  Patchy sclerotic bone and subperiosteal bone formation at the upper end of the left humerus.

2  Chronic osteomyelitis.

3  It most commonly occurs as a sequel to acute osteomyelitis associated with an open fracture.

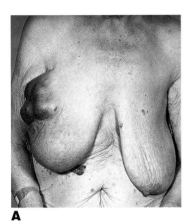

**A**

1 What is the diagnosis?

2 What are the characteristics of this lesion?

3 How does this tumour spread?

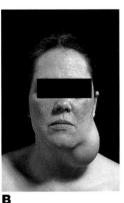

**B**

1 What is the differential diagnosis of this cystic lesion?

2 Excision revealed a squamous epithelial lining. What is the diagnosis?

3 What is the aetiology of this lesion?

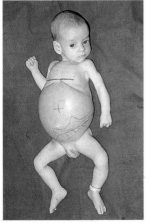

**C**

1 This baby has a Wilms' tumour (nephroblastoma). What type of tumour is this?

2 What clinical features may there be?

3 What other congenital abnormalities are associated with this tumour?

# Answers page 73

## A

1 Brodie's cystosarcoma phyllodes of the right breast.

2 Uneven consistency and a bosselated surface. The breast may be tense and firm, with thin skin and enlarged veins. Occasionally there is ulceration over the base of the tumour, which may present as a fungating mass.

3 The tumour spreads locally, enlarging to a considerable size. Fixation to the skin or deep structures is uncommon and a late feature of the disease: only rarely is there spread to lymph nodes or distant metastases.

## B

1 (a) Branchial cyst
  (b) TB abscess.

2 Branchial cyst.

3 It is a congenital anomaly from the remnant of ectodermal placodes from the first, second or fourth branchial cleft.

## C

1 This is an embryonic tumour. It accounts for 11–13 per cent of childhood tumours. Five to ten per cent of Wilms' tumours are bilateral.

2 Usually an abdominal mass with signs of weight loss. Occasionally the child may have a pyrexia and haematuria.

3 Hypospadias, non-familial aniridia, hemihypertrophy of the body, Beckwith–Weidemann syndrome (exophthalmos, macroglossia and gigantism).

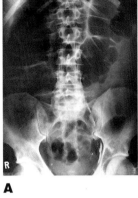

**A**

1  What does this radiograph show?

2  What is the probable diagnosis?

3  What are the poor prognostic features of this condition?

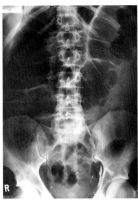

**B**

1  Histology of this lesion revealed Reed–Sternberg cells: what is the diagnosis?

2  What are the aetiological factors of the disease?

3  What are the stages of the disease?

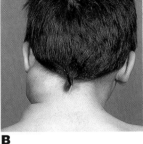

**C**

1  Describe this lesion.

2  What is the diagnosis?

3  What are the predisposing factors?

# Answers page 75

## A

1 Toxic megacolon.

2 Inflammatory bowel disease, uncontrolled exacerbated ulcerative colitis.

3 A severe initial attack, late onset disease and involvement of the whole colon.

## B

1 Hodgkin's lymphoma.

2 The disease occurs in young adults and may be associated with chromosomal abnormalities and infection with the Epstein–Barr virus.

3 Ann Arbor staging:
   - I – single node region or extralymphatic site
   - II – two or more node regions on the same side of the diaphragm or single node region and one extralymphatic site on one side of the diaphragm
   - III – node regions on both sides of the diaphragm
   - IV – diffuse involvement of one or more extralymphatic sites.

## C

1 Necrotic ulceration of the cheek, with black slough of the skin.

2 Cancrum oris.

3 Caused in malnourished children by measles, gastroentertitis, typhoid, bronchopneumonia and kala-azar.

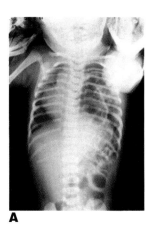

**A**

1 What is the abnormality in this radiograph?

2 What is the differential diagnosis?

3 How does it present?

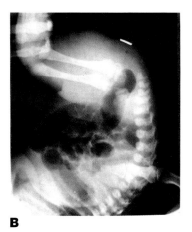

**B**

1 Describe this figure.

2 What is the most likely diagnosis?

3 What are the various types of this abnormality?

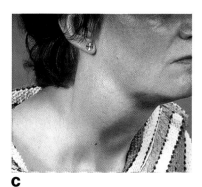

**C**

This figure shows a woman with a carotid body tumour.

1 From where do these tumours originate?

2 In what group of people is this tumour found?

3 How may these patients present?

# Answers page 77

## A

1  The left hemithorax is filled with abdominal contents and the mediastinum is shifted to the right.

2  Diaphragmatic hernia, either of Bochdalek or Morgagni type. These are congenital. They may also be due to a diaphragmatic rupture.

3  There is gradual, increasing respiratory distress.

## B

1  Radiograph taken of a child in an inverted (head down) position in order to fill the rectum with air. A coin marker is placed over the anus.

2  Imperforate anus.

3  High – the bowel ending above or at the level of the pelvic floor; low – the bowel ending below the pelvic floor.

## C

1  Carotid body tumours are chemodectomas and arise from the chemoreceptor cells of the carotid body. They form part of a group of neuroendocrine tumours, e.g. phaeochromocytomas and paraganglionomas.

2  They occur more often in people living at high altitude, where carotid body hyperplasia results from long-standing hypoxaemia. There is an autosomal dominant genetic tendency which may account for bilateral cases.

3  Carotid body tumours present as a painless lump in the neck, generally in the 40–50-year age group. In 10 per cent of cases there may be localized nerve damage resulting in palsies of the 7th to 12th cranial nerves. On rare occasions invasion of the carotid arteries can produce transient ischaemic neurological symptoms. On examination the tumour is a hard, regular mass at the carotid bifurcation. It exhibits transmitted pulsation and, owing to its relationship with the carotid artery, the tumour may be moved horizontally but has very little vertical mobility.

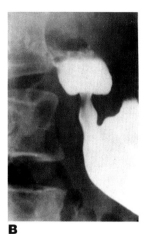

**A**

1  What is the diagnosis?
2  What are the clinical features of this disease?
3  What is its aetiology?

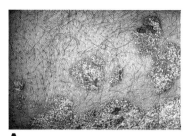

**B**

1  What does this radiograph show?
2  How may this condition present?
3  What are the causes of this condition?
4  In children with this condition, what other features are often present?

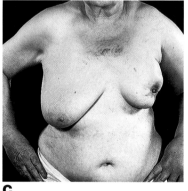

**C**

1  What does this figure show?
2  What is the effect of pressing the hands on the hips?

# Answers page 79

## A

1  Psoriasis.

2  Clinically this disease involves skin, nails and bone.

   (a) Skin: typically the skin lesions in psoriasis are well-demarcated, salmon pink, topped with silver scale. The vast majority of patients have lesions over extensor surfaces, eyes, knees and elbows, with scattered smaller lesions over the limbs. Scalp involvement is also common

   (b) nails: this can occur in isolation or in combination with skin lesions. The changes most commonly seen are pitting and onycholysis

   (c) bone: this is a sero-negative arthritis occurring in 10 per cent of patients with psoriasis. Commonly this presents as a polyarthritis, involving the small joints of the hands. There is also an increased incidence of ankylosing spondylitis in these patients.

3  (a) Genetic factors: the mode of inheritance of psoriasis is not known, although there is an increased incidence in people with HLAB13 and B17. HLAB27 is also seen in patients with ankylosing spondylitis and spinal arthropathy

   (b) infection: in children guttate psoriasis occurs ten to fourteen days after a throat infection with a beta haemolytic Streptococcus

   (c) drugs: lithium carbonate and beta antagonists may exacerbate psoriasis

   (d) emotional trauma: an increased incidence of psoriasis is seen during times of great stress, e.g. examinations.

## B

1  Hypertrophic pyloric stenosis.

2  Patients present with symptoms and signs of gastric outflow obstruction, i.e. abdominal distension, fullness and discomfort and profuse vomiting containing old, undigested food. Peristaltic waves may be seen and a succussion splash may be heard.

3  Pyloric stenosis may be congenital or acquired. Acquired causes include:
   (a) fibrosis secondary to chronic distal gastric or proximal duodenal ulceration;
   (b) gastric or duodenal malignancy; (c) external compression from malignancy in adjacent organs.

4  This condition is associated with a male predominance (1:4), is often found in the first-born and the child usually has affected siblings or parents.

## C

1  Left breast cancer, puckered by the patient pressing her hands on her hips.

2  Pressing the hands on the hips tenses the pectoralis major muscle and demonstrates the fixity of overlying pathology.

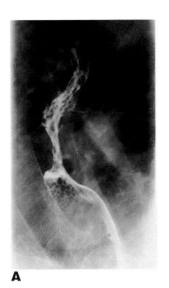

**A**

1 What does this barium swallow show?

2 What are the risk factors for developing this condition?

3 What options are available for palliative treatment?

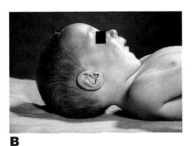

**B**

1 What does this figure show?

2 What are the differential diagnoses?

3 What condition is characterized by fibrous dysplasia of the maxilla and ethmoid bones?

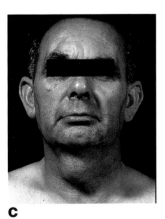

**C**

1 What is the most likely diagnosis?

2 What is the embryology of this lesion?

3 How may this be differentiated from a thyroid mass?

# Answers page 81

## A

1  A carcinoma of the middle third of the oesophagus. This is a malignant stricture.

2  Smoking, high alcohol intake, lye strictures, nitrosamines in the diet, achalasia, Plummer–Vinson syndrome, Barrett's oesophagus.

3  The malignant stricture can be intubated under direct vision. The lesion can be bypassed with the stomach (Kirschner's operation) or partially resected: both procedures carry a high mortality. Laser therapy can decrease tumour regrowth by fibrosis but initially has to be carried out repeatedly.

## B

1  Micrognathia; shortened horizontal ramus of the mandible; facial abnormalities.

2  Pierre Robin, Crouzen's and Apert's syndromes.

3  Albright's syndrome with facial abnormalities.

## C

1  Infrahyoid thyroglossal cyst.

2  The thyroid develops from a cell mass arising at the base of the tongue and descends in the mid-line of the neck to lie anterior to the third and fourth tracheal rings. The line of descent of the thyroglossal tract therefore extends from the foramen caecum of the tongue to the isthmus of the thyroid gland. If part of the tract fails to atrophy after full descent of the thyroid gland a thyroglossal cyst is formed; 90 per cent lie in front of the hyoid bone, 8 per cent below and 2 per cent lingually.

3  Both thyroglossal cysts and thyroid masses move upwards on swallowing but a thyroglossal cyst also moves upwards on protrusion of the tongue.

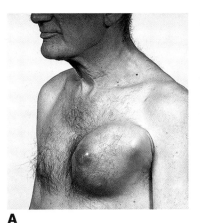

**A**

1 What is this lesion?
2 What is its incidence?
3 How does it present?

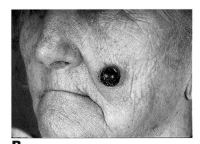

**B**

1 What is the diagnosis?
2 What are the clinical features?
3 Where are the common sites for this lesion?

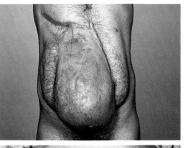

**C**

1 Describe these figures.
2 What are the causes of these lesions?
3 What are the common complications?

# Answers page 83

## A

1  Carcinoma of the male breast.

2  Less than 1 per cent of breast carcinomas.

3  It presents as a lump, as in the female breast, but may be ignored. Fixation to skin and underlying muscle is an earlier manifestation than in the female owing to reduced fat content.

## B

1  Pigmented lesion on the left cheek of an old lady, probably a malignant melanoma.

2  A dark polypoid mass (it may be pale), variable degrees of invasion, there may be metastatic involvement of local or distant nodes and of other organs.

3  It may occur in any part of the face, as well as in the nasal septum or lateral wall of the nose. Common sites are on the limbs, particularly exposed surfaces.

## C

1  Huge incisional herniae through old operation scars.

2  Obesity and infection are the two main causes. Other precipitating factors include hypertension, cardiac and renal disorders, diabetes and jaundice.

3  Irreducibility is common but strangulation unusual, unless the neck of the sac is very small.

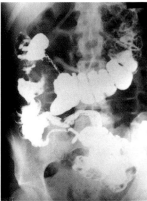

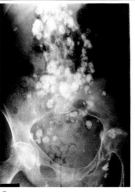

A

1 What are the intestinal types of this inflammatory lesion?

2 What is the differential diagnosis?

3 How would you assess this patient?

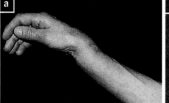

B

1 What is the most likely diagnosis?

2 What is the causative organism?

3 What toxin is produced by the micro-organism?

4 What are the systemic symptoms?

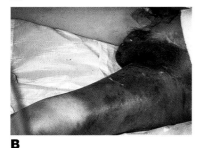

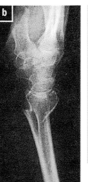

C

1 Describe figure (a).

2 Describe radiograph (b).

3 What is the major immediate complication?

4 What are the commonest late complications?

# Answers page 85

## A

1 Tuberculous enteritis presents with ulcerative, hypertrophic, ulcerohypertrophic, ascitic or fibrotic lesions.

2 Crohn's disease, postoperative stricture and benign and malignant tumours.

3 History of pulmonary TB and signs of anaemia and malnutrition. Investigation by Mantoux test, chest radiographs. Exclude other diseases by general stool examinations, e.g. Salmonella, Shigella and Yersinia, pseudomembraneous colitis.

## B

1 Gas gangrene of the upper thigh.

2 *Clostridium perfringens/welchii.*

3 Exotoxin.

4 Shock, crepitus, bluish-brown skin discoloration, bullous formation with a watery discharge and a pronounced odour. The fluid from the bullae provides a heavy growth of the causative organism.

## C

1 'Dinner fork' deformity, typically seen in a Colles' fracture.

2 A distal fracture of the radius with dorsal shifting of the distal fragment, dorsal angulation and radial shift.

3 Median nerve compression from direct pressure.

4 Malunion, rupture of the extensor pollicis longus tendon, osteoarthritis of the wrist joint, Sudeck's osteodystrophy and chronic pain.

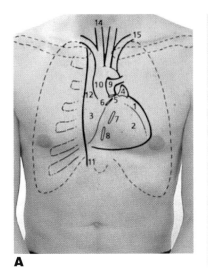

**A**

1  What are these markings?

2  Label 4, 5, 7, 9 and 14.

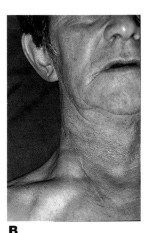

**B**

1  What is the diagnosis in this patient, who has recently been found to have malignant cells in his sputum?

2  What is the significance of supraclavicular lymphadenopathy?

3  What is the significance of left supraclavicular involvement?

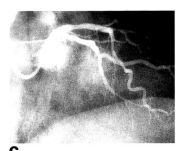

**C**

1  What does this arteriogram show?

2  What symptoms may be present?

3  What is the differential diagnosis of anginal pain?

# Answers page 87

## A

1  Surface markings of the heart and great vessels.

2  4 – left atrial appendage; 5 – pulmonary valve; 7 – mitral valve; 9 – pulmonary trunk; 14 – right common carotid artery.

## B

1  Supraclavicular malignant lymph node secondary to carcinoma of the lung.

2  In cervical lymphadenopathy, primary head and neck carcinomas should be excluded. The great exception to this rule is the supraclavicular fossa, where three-quarters of the associated primary tumours are infraclavicular in origin.

3  Isolated left supraclavicular lymphadenopathy may result from spread along the thoracic duct from gastric or pancreatic carcinomas (Troisier's sign: Virchow's node).

## C

1  Stenosis at the bifurcation of the left coronary artery.

2  Typically, patients with angina present with substernal pain, which is often described as 'gripping' in nature. The pain may radiate to the arm, jaws or neck. Generally it is exacerbated by exercise but in a patient with unstable angina it may come on at rest. Myocardial infarction presents with constant pain in the same distribution.

3  Acute dissection of a thoracic aortic aneurysm, pleuritic chest pain secondary to pneumonia, pulmonary embolus, cholecystitis.

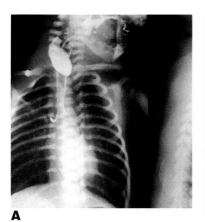

**A**

1 What does this figure show?

2 What are the common anatomical variants of this condition?

3 How may these children present?

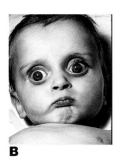

**B**

1 Describe the appearance of this baby with diarrhoea.

2 What are the signs of dehydration?

3 What are the principles of management?

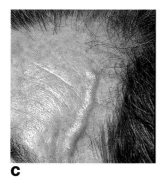

**C**

1 What is the diagnosis?

2 What is the pathology behind this disease?

3 How may this disease present?

4 How is the diagnosis made?

# Answers page 89

## A

1   Oesophageal atresia with a tracheal fistula.

2   Eighty-five per cent of oesophageal atresias have a proximal blind ending pouch of oesophagus whereas the distal oesophagus connects to the trachea. In 12 per cent there is a proximal blind ending oesophagus and no connection of the distal oesophagus to trachea. In 2 per cent the proximal oesophagus is connected to the trachea, whereas the distal oesophagus is not. In 1 per cent of cases both the proximal and distal oesophagus are connected to the trachea.

3   The pathognomonic sign is profuse, foaming saliva flowing from the mouth and nostrils. Feeding is always associated with coughing and if the feed enters the lung an inhalation pneumonia may develop. Oesophageal atresia should also be suspected in babies who have polyhydramnios.

## B

1   Severe dehydration, with sunken eyes.

2   Reduced skin turgor, oliguria, tachycardia and hypotension, low CVP/JVP, lethargy, depressed fontanelles.

3   The degree of dehydration is precisely assessed and rehydration and resuscitation undertaken. Fluid replacement is according to the daily requirement, additional fluid losses and correction of deficit.

## C

1   Temporal arteritis.

2   This is a granulomatous arteritis of unknown aetiology, affecting mainly the over-sixties and usually involving the extracranial arteries. Histologically there is inflammation of the full thickness of the affected arteries. The vessel wall is involved in a granulomatous reaction, with an accumulation of lymphocytes, macrophages and Langhans' giant cells (hence the alternative name of giant cell arteritis).

3   (a) Headache felt over the inflamed, superficial temporal artery. The arterial pulsation is soon lost and the artery feels tortuous and thickened
   (b) facial pain. Pain in the face, mouth and jaw occurs, caused by inflammation of the facial, maxillary and lingual branches of the external carotid artery. The pain is characteristically worse on eating

   (c) visual problems. Visual loss may occur in 25 per cent of untreated cases owing to inflammation or occlusion of the ciliary or central retinal artery. The patient may complain of sudden, uniocular visual loss

4   The diagnosis is made clinically and confirmed by a high ESR and histologically by a temporal artery biopsy.

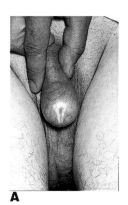

**A**

1 What is the diagnosis?
2 What are the causes?
3 What is the treatment?

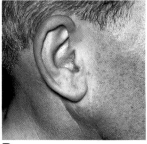

**B**

1 What does this figure show?
2 What are the differential diagnoses of this condition?
3 What are the commonest tumours in this area?
4 How can you distinguish clinically between benign and malignant salivary gland tumours?

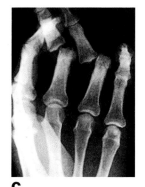

**C**

1 Describe this radiograph.
2 How would this patient present?
3 What are the commonest complications?

# Answers page 91

## A

1  Phimosis.

2  Chronic balanitis in the elderly (this may indicate diabetes). Balanitis xerotica obliterans in 20- to 40-year-old men, balanoprosthitis in children and congenital pin-hole opening of the foreskin.

3  In children sometimes just the prepucial adhesions need to be excised, but the usual treatment is formal circumcision.

## B

1  Unilateral parotid swelling.

2  (a)Swelling of the parotid gland itself: parotitis, mixed parotid tumour or adenolymphoma, carcinoma
   (b)swelling of other anatomical structures in the vicinity: sebaceous cyst, lipoma, enlarged pre-auricular or parotid lymph nodes, neuroma of the facial nerve, mandibular swelling or tumour.

3  Pleomorphic adenoma (mixed parotid tumour), adenolymphoma (Warthin's tumour).

4  Typically malignant tumours produce indistinct, rapidly growing masses, associated with cervical lymphadenopathy. They are usually hard, fixed masses and may be associated with localized pain, referred otalgia and nerve palsies. Facial nerve palsy may occur with a malignant parotid tumour. Infiltration of the lingual nerve may occur in malignant tumours of the submandibular gland, producing numbness of the anterior two-thirds of the tongue.

## C

1  Scaphoid fracture with proximal sclerosis from avascular necrosis.

2  The fracture usually occurs in young adults after falling on the outstretched hand; there is pain and tenderness in the anatomical snuffbox, which can be easily missed. The diagnosis can be confirmed radiologically with scaphoid views. Suspicious cases should be immobilized in a scaphoid cast and the radiology reviewed after two weeks.

3  Non-union, avascular necrosis of the proximal pole.

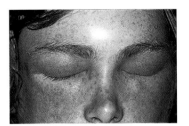

**A**

1 What does this figure show?
2 What are the causes?

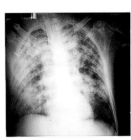

**B**

1 Describe this chest radiograph of a 38-year-old man who presented with severe respiratory distress eight days after sustaining eight rib fractures and a fracture of the upper end of the humerus.
2 What is the diagnosis?
3 What are the causes of this condition?

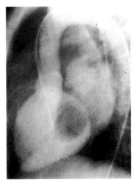

**C**

1 What does this radiograph show?
2 Where is this lesion most commonly found?
3 How may this patient present?
4 What physical signs are usually present?

# Answers page 93

## A

1   Oedematous swelling of the eyelids and forehead owing to acute or chronic frontal sinusitis.

2   Osteomyelitis of frontal sinuses, Pott's puffy tumour, orbital cellulitis with possible sub-orbital abscess, intracranial infection, thrombophlebitis of the cavernous or sagittal sinuses or cerebral abscess.

## B

1   Widespread bilateral diffuse interstitial pulmonary shadowing.

2   Shock injury or adult respiratory distress syndrome.

3   Trauma, shock, sepsis, pancreatitis, obstetric complications, coagulopathy, tumours.

## C

1   Atrial myxoma.

2   Atrial myxomas usually develop in the left atrium. It is a polypoid, gelatinous structure attached by a pedicle to the atrial septum. Myxomas also occur in the right atrium or the ventricles but are much rarer.

3   The myxoma may obstruct the mitral valve or be a site of thrombi which can then embolize, giving rise to peripheral ischaemic symptoms. The patient may also present with shortness of breath, syncope and a mild fever.

4   A mild first heart sound, a tumour plop (loud third heart sound as a pedunculated tumour comes to an abrupt halt), a mid-diastolic murmur and signs resulting from embolization.

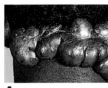

**A**

1 What is the diagnosis?

2 What is the composition of this lesion?

3 Which sites would you most expect to be involved?

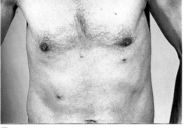

**B**

1 What is this anomaly?

2 Where may it occur?

3 Name three other congenital abnormalities of the breast.

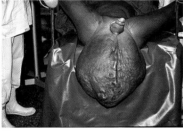

**C**

1 What is the diagnosis?

2 What are the causes?

3 What complications may occur?

# Answers page 95

## A

1  Keloid scar.

2  Hyperplastic vascular collagen fibres which can extend in a claw-like fashion into adjacent tissues for a number of years. It is common in individuals with pigmented skin, in children, in pregnancy and it may be familial.

3  Keloid is most commonly distributed in the midline, over the face, the neck, the sternum, arms and anterior abdominal wall. It can be copious after a burn, radiotherapy and even after a BCG inoculation.

## B

1  Accessory nipple.

2  It is sited in a line from the axilla to the groin, i.e. along the milk line.

3  Amastia, hypoplasia of the breast, hyperplasia of the breast.

## C

1  Elephantiasis of the scrotum.

2  Tuberculosis lymphadenitis is the commonest cause. Chronic sepsis and filariasis.

3  Recurrent sepsis and, rarely, the development of a lymphangiosarcoma.

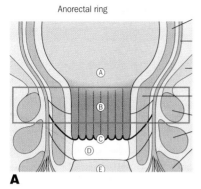

**A**

In this diagram of the anal canal and anal sphincter:

1 To what does the blue line refer?

2 To what does B refer?

3 To what does C refer?

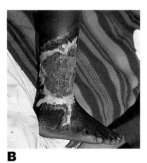

**B**

1 Describe this lesion.

2 What is the differential diagnosis?

3 What are the commonest causative micro-organisms?

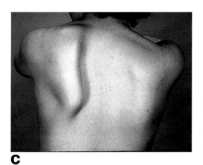

**C**

1 What does this figure show?

2 What is the cause?

3 What is the commonest iatrogenic cause?

# Answers page 97

## A

1  The anorectal ring.

2  The anal mucosa and anal venous columns.

3  The dentate line.

## B

1  An ulcer with undermined edge and a zone of skin in the immediate vicinity is infiltrated and raised. There is copious serosanguinous discharge.

2  Tropical ulcer, yaws, Veld sore, Buruli ulcer, venous ulcer, malignant melanoma.

3  *Fusobacterium fusiformis, Borrelia vincenti.*

## C

1  Winging of the left scapula.

2  Injury to the accessory or long thoracic nerves.

3  Damage resulting from surgical excision during lymph node biopsy in the posterior triangle of the neck, or from axillary clearance in breast cancer surgery.

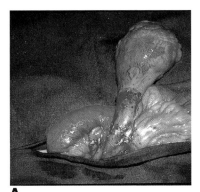

**A**

1 What does this figure show?

2 What is the embryology of this lesion?

3 Where is this classically found?

4 How may this patient present?

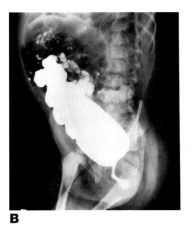

**B**

1 What does this radiograph show?

2 What is the pathophysiology of this disease?

3 What is its natural history?

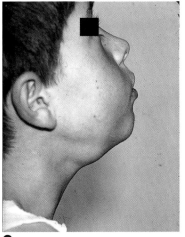

**C**

1 What does this figure show?

2 What are the possible causes of this condition?

3 How may submandibular sialolithiasis present?

4 What structures are at risk during the excision of a submandibular gland?

# Answers page 99

## A

1  Meckel's diverticulum.

2  It is a remnant of the vitellointestinal duct.

3  Two feet from the ileocaecal valve, classically in 2 per cent of the population and is two inches long.

4  A Meckel's diverticulum may be: (a) asymptomatic; (b) inflamed, mimicking acute appendicitis; (c) it may be an apex of an intussusception or the site of an umbilical band, causing intestinal obstruction or volvulus; (d) it may also contain gastric mucosa, which is subject to ulceration, haemorrhage and perforation.

## B

1  Hirschsprung's disease.

2  It is due to failure of the myenteric plexus of the bowel to migrate, thus leading to aganglionosis of the bowel. The condition always starts at the distal rectum but may spread into the small intestine. Inability of the bowel to perform peristalsis leads to constipation. Hirschsprung's disease is the commonest cause of intestinal obstruction in the newborn. It has a 4:1 male predominance, and 90 per cent of cases present in the first three days of life.

3  Most cases present in the neonatal period, although occasionally the condition may not be diagnosed until adulthood, when there is a history of life-long constipation. The history is of a neonate unable to pass meconium in the first two to three days of life. Meconium is usually passed after the passage of a finger into the rectum. Constipation then returns. The abdomen becomes increasingly distended and the proximal colon becomes increasingly enlarged, forming a megacolon, and may perforate.

## C

1  Submandibular gland swelling.

2  (a)  Sialolithiasis
   (b)  malignancy - carcinomas, primary or rarely secondary
   (c)  infection, e.g. viral (mumps), bacterial
   (d)  autoimmune disorders, e.g. Mikulicz's or Sjögren's syndromes.

3  Pain and swelling of the gland on eating – swelling subsides over the next hour. Occasionally the stone may be palpated in Wharton's duct from inside the oral cavity.

4  (a)  Mandibular branch of the facial nerve
   (b)  hypoglossal nerve
   (c)  lingual nerve.

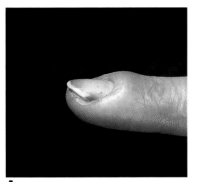

A

1 What is the diagnosis?
2 What is the causative organism?

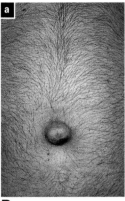

B

1 What is this umbilical swelling?
2 What is the classification of this swelling?
3 State the causative factors in the development of umbilical and para-umbilical herniae.

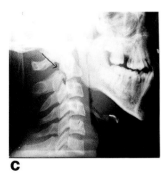

C

1 What does this radiograph show?
2 How would this patient present?
3 How should the patient be examined?

# Answers page 101

## A

1  Chronic paronychia.

2  Chronic inflammation, either owing to bacterial infection (Streptococcus or Staphylococcus) or secondary to fungal infection, such as candidiasis.

## B

1  Umbilical hernia.

2  They are congenital or acquired. Most adult herniae are acquired and are really para-umbilical, in which about half the fundus of the sac is covered by the umbilicus and the remainder by the adjacent abdominal skin.

3  An umbilical hernia is congenital and is precipitated by a chronic increase in intra-abdominal pressure; para-umbilical herniae are more common in multiparous women and obese patients.

## C

1  Unstable fracture of the 2nd cervical vertebra.

2  In the unconscious patient, flaccid areflexia, diaphragmatic breathing, hypotension with bradycardia, neurogenic shock and priapism all suggest a spinal cord injury. In the conscious patient, joint pains in the cervical vertebrae with neck pain and severe tenderness.

3  The patient is examined in a neutral position, with the neck held immobilized in line immobilization or stabilized with a collar and sandbags. To assess the back of the spine the patient is log-rolled. This requires at least one person to control the head, two to hold the pelvis and trunk and one to examine the back.

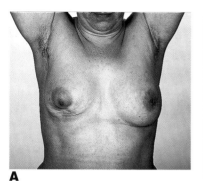

1  What does this figure show?

2  What is the effect of arm elevation?

3  What is the usual pathological finding with this skin change?

**A**

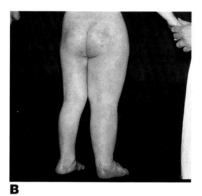

1  What are the differential diagnoses of gigantism of the right lower limb?

2  How would you investigate lymphoedema?

3  What treatment options are available for lymphoedema?

**B**

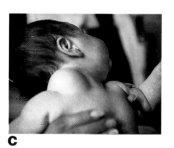

1  What is this condition?

2  What is its pathology?

3  What clinical signs can usually be demonstrated in this lesion?

4  How is the condition managed?

**C**

# Answers page 103

## A

1  Arm elevation showing skin tethering from an underlying neoplasm.

2  Lumps that are large in comparison with the size of the breast may be evident on first inspection; further abnormalities may become evident when the arms are moved.

3  Neoplastic infiltration.

## B

1  Unilateral enlargement of all tissues suggests an arteriovenous malformation, as in this patient, but always remember the abnormality may be hypoplasia of the contralateral limb. Gross subcutaneous enlargement is usually primary or secondary lymphoedema but venous oedema, owing to obstruction and thrombosis, may be marked.

2  Exclude all other causes. Proceed to lymphography and radionuclide lymphatic clearance studies.

3  Over 90 per cent of patients can be treated conservatively, with compression stockings, intermittent pneumatic compression and early prevention or treatment of any infections which may develop. The remainder need surgery. De-bulking operations, such as Homan's operation, aim to remove the subcutaneous tissue. Lymph drainage procedures involve lymphovenous shunts or bridging operations.

## C

1  Cystic hygroma.

2  Cystic hygromas are subcutaneous, multilocular, non-communicating lymph channels. They tend to occur in babies, particularly in the neck, groins and axillae.

3  Fluctuance and brilliant transillumination.

4  The management is conservative and most lesions resolve spontaneously by the age of four years. Aspiration and injection with sclerosants may be required for persistent lesions.

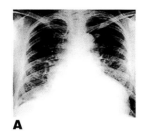

**A**

1　Describe the radiological findings.

2　What are the likely symptoms in this patient?

3　What are the predisposing factors for developing this disease?

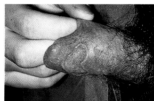

**B**

1　What is this condition?

2　How does it present?

3　What is its treatment?

4　What are the indications for circumcision?

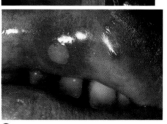

**C**

1　What abnormalities are present in these figures?

2　What is the likely diagnosis?

3　What other conditions are associated with oral ulceration?

# Answers page 105

## A

1 Enlarged heart, enlargement of the pulmonary conus and increased pulmonary vascular marking.

2 An elderly male smoker with marked dyspnoea, orthopnoea, paroxysmal nocturnal dyspnoea and a productive cough.

3 Obesity, smoking, hypertension, myocardial disease, e.g. myocardial infarction, cardiomyopathies.

## B

1 Balanitis xerotica obliterans (also known as lichen sclerosis et atrophicus).

2 Urinary symptoms secondary to meatal stenosis or with a phimosis.

3 Circumcision.

4 Other indications for circumcision include religious or social grounds, phimosis or paraphimosis, recurrent balanitis (especially in diabetics) and as a prelude to radiotherapy for carcinoma of the penis.

## C

1 Oral and penile ulceration.

2 Behçet's syndrome: a disease of unknown immunological origin, which presents with oral and genital ulceration, uveitis, arthritis, transient neurological symptoms and thrombosis.

3 HIV, other immunosuppressed states, e.g. leucopenic, neutropenia, infection with herpes simplex and cytomegalovirus, and aphthous ulceration.
   ● Bacterial infections include Vincent's angina, cancrum oris, TB and syphilis.
   ● Fungal infections.
   ● Trauma, e.g. toothbrush or dentures.
   ● Metal poisoning, e.g. lead, gold, bismuth and mercury.
   ● Drugs, particularly phenytoin and antiviral drugs: more extreme cases can produce Stevens–Johnson syndrome.
   ● Other causes of oral ulceration include pemphigus and pemphigoid, other autoimmune diseases, leucoplakia, scurvy and pellagra, Crohn's and ulcerative colitis.

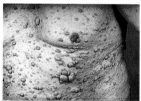

**A**

1  What is this condition?
2  From what does this develop?
3  What is its lining?
4  What are its anatomical relationships?

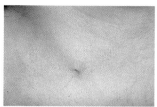

**B**

1  What is the diagnosis?
2  How is it inherited?
3  What other skin lesions are associated with this disease?
4  What other abnormalities are associated with this condition?

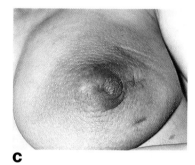

**C**

1  What is this lesion?
2  What are the common causes?
3  What is important in the management of a persistent lesion?

# Answers page 107

## A

1 Branchial fistula.

2 A branchial fistula develops from a persistent branchial cleft (usually second or fourth). They are usually congenital but may be acquired following excision of a branchial cyst.

3 Stratified squamous epithelium.

4 Branchial fistulae present at or soon after birth as a discharging orifice on the anterior aspect of the neck. The orifice usually lies at the anterior border of the sternocleidomastoid muscle. A fistulous tract passes from the skin, between the internal and external carotid arteries, superior to the hypoglossal nerve, inferior to the glossopharyngeal nerve, to open into the tonsillar fossa.

## B

1 Multiple neurofibromatoses.

2 Autosomal dominant.

3 Café-au-lait patches and fibroepithelial skin tags.

4 Neural tumours, e.g. ganglioneuromas, phaeochromocytomas, gliomas, meningiomas, bilateral spinal and acoustic neuromas, scoliosis, renal artery stenosis, pulmonary fibrosis and orbital haemangiomas.

## C

1 Oedema and inflammation of the right breast from an underlying abscess.

2 Most infections of the breast follow trauma, the commonest of which is breast feeding. Infections can also occur in the glands of Montgomery, giving rise to subareolar mastitis.

3 When the history is prolonged, without marked tenderness and there is generalized induration, mastitis carcinomatosa, a rapidly advancing carcinoma, should be excluded.

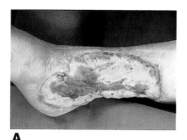

**A**

1  What is the diagnosis?
2  What is this type of ulcer known as?
3  How may this be treated?

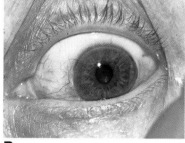

**B**

1  What is the lesion shown in this figure?
2  What is the cause?
3  What are the symptoms?

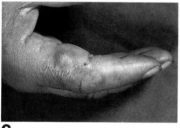

**C**

1  What is the diagnosis in this butcher who denied any history of trauma?
2  What is the causative organism?
3  What is the source of the infection?

# Answers page 109

## A

1  Malignant change in a chronic venous ulcer.

2  Marjolin's ulcer.

3  Usually local excision and / or radiotherapy. However, in this case a below-knee amputation may be the only option. Regional lymph node involvement is treated by surgical block dissection.

## B

1  Calcified band around the periphery of the cornea.

2  Hypercalcaemia.

3  Anorexia, vomiting, polyuria, polydypsia, abdominal pain, renal stones, pruritus, psychiatric problems (depression), ECG changes (prolongation of QT interval).

## C

1  Erysipeloid infection.

2  *Erysipelothrix* sp. bacteria.

3  Contaminated meat, game or fish.

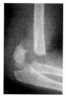

**A**

1  Describe this radiograph.
2  What is the most serious complication?

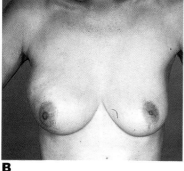

**B**

1  What abnormality is present in this figure?
2  Which common benign breast lesions present as a lump?

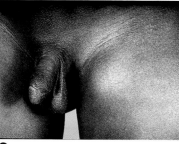

**C**

1  What is the most likely diagnosis in this boy with a history of a cat bite two weeks previously?
2  What sites are most commonly affected?
3  What findings would support the diagnosis?

# Answers page 111

## A

1  Supracondylar fracture of the humerus, angulated and tilted dorsally.

2  Ischaemia of the forearm and hand which, if left untreated, will give rise to a Volkmann's contracture.

## B

1  There is a symmetrical swelling in the right upper quadrant of the right breast.

2  Cysts, aberration of normal growth and development, fibroadenoma, acute or chronic infection, fat necrosis, galactocele.

## C

1  Left inguinal lymphadenopathy from cat scratch disease.

2  The axillary and inguinal nodes are almost exclusively affected.

3  An enlarged spleen and confirmation by specific intradermal testing or node biopsy.

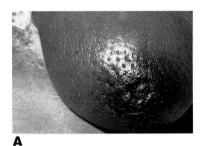

**A**

1 What does this figure show?
2 What is the pathophysiology of this condition?
3 What is the cause of this condition?

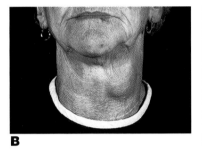

**B**

1 What does this figure show?
2 What are the differential diagnoses of this condition?
3 How should this patient be investigated?

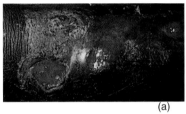

(a)

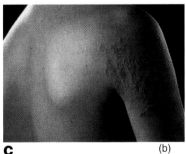

**C**   (b)

1 What is the causative agent in both of these figures?
2 Describe the lesion shown in figure (a)?
3 What is the cause of the lesion shown in figure (b)?

# Answers page 113

## A

1  Peau d'orange.

2  Infiltration of the lymphatic drainage of the breast gives rise to cutaneous oedema. The tiny pits are produced by deep tethering of the sweat glands.

3  Breast neoplasia is the commonest cause but peau d'orange may also be secondary to chronic inflammation of the breast, e.g. chronic intramammary abscesses.

## B

1  Solitary nodule in the left lobe of the thyroid.

2  Multinodular goitre – 50 per cent of solitary nodules are part of a multinodular goitre; haemorrhage into or necrosis of a hyperplastic nodule; adenoma, carcinoma (papillary, follicular), enlargement of the whole lobe secondary to thyroiditis.

3  Ultrasound scanning should be performed to confirm the solitary nature of the nodule (since this may be part of a multinodular goitre) and to determine whether it is cystic or solid. Fine needle aspiration should be performed. If fluid is aspirated from a cyst, and it does not recur, no further treatment is necessary. If repeated fine needle aspiration indicates benign disease, no surgical intervention is necessary unless symptoms determine otherwise. If fine needle aspiration indicates follicular or papillary cells, surgical resection is necessary.

## C

1  Guinea worm (*Dracunculus medinensis*).

2  Extensive skin inflammation and ulceration following guinea worm infection.

3  Cutaneous larvae migrans.

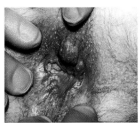

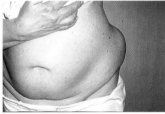

**A**

1  What does this figure show?

2  In what positions are these lesions commonly found?

3  How may these patients present?

4  What is a sentinel pile?

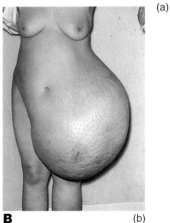

(a)

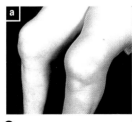

**B**          (b)

1  What is the common site of both pathologies?

2  What does figure (a) show?

3  What does figure (b) show?

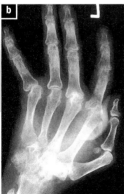

**C**

1  Describe figure (a).

2  Describe the radiographic abnormalities in figure (b).

3  What is the diagnosis common to both figures?

4  What associated signs may be present?

# Answers page 115

## A

1 Anal fissure.

2 Anal fissures are almost always midline; 90 per cent are posterior in men but a higher proportion (approximately 20 per cent) are anterior in women.

3 Patients typically present with pain immediately after defaecation. Bright red blood is seen on the toilet paper and a stinging sensation often accompanies wiping. Many patients also suffer from pruritus ani.

4 A sentinel pile occurs with a chronic anal fissure, where the skin of the lower part of the fissure becomes swollen. This may be the only sign of the fissure, as it is often too painful to examine the patient proctoscopically.

## B

1 The common site of both pathologies is the abdominal wall.

2 Lipoma of the left side of the lower abdomen.

3 A benign leiomyoma.

## C

1 Swelling of both knee joints, with effusion and quadriceps atrophy.

2 Joint destruction of the metacarpophalangeal joints, enlarged joints, ulnar deviation.

3 Rheumatoid arthritis.

4 Widespread deformity and rheumatoid nodules. Extra-articular features of the disease include pericarditis and pulmonary abnormalities such as pleurisy, pulmonary nodules and fibrosis.

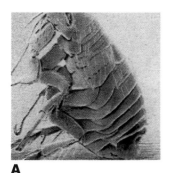

**A**

1   What does this figure show?
2   What is its medical significance?

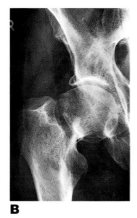

**B**

1   What is the site of the lesion demonstrated in this radiograph?
2   How is this fracture classified?
3   What is the major factor in the healing of such a fracture?

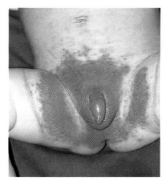

**C**

1   Describe this figure.
2   What does it show?
3   What is the cause?

# Answers page 117

## A

1  A flea.

2  There are more than twenty species of flea that attack humans; the commonest variety in the UK is *Pulex irritans*. It causes irritation and erythema.

## B

1  Intracapsular fracture of the neck of the right femur.

2  A fracture of the neck of the femur is either intracapsular (subcapital or cervical) or extracapsular (basicervical or intertrochanteric).

3  The major factor influencing healing is the blood supply to the femoral head. If this is compromised, most commonly occurring in an intracapsular fracture in an elderly patient, non-union and avascular necrosis can result.

## C

1  Erythematous skin changes involving genitalia, buttocks and around the anal orifice.

2  Nappy rash.

3  It arises because of prolonged contact with urine or faeces but may also be due to fungal infection or reaction to an emollient.

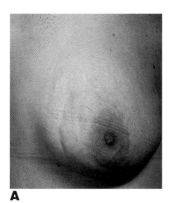

**A**

1   What does this figure show?

2   What causes this condition?

3   What is its significance?

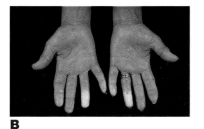

**B**

1   What is the diagnosis?

2   What conditions may predispose to this condition?

3   What are the physiological mechanisms behind this syndrome?

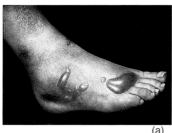

(a)

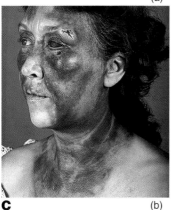

**C**                                        (b)

1   What do these figures show?

2   What other immediate complications might there be?

3   What is the characteristic feature in figure (a)

# Answers page 119

## A

1 Superficial phlebitis or Mondor's disease.

2 Venous engorgement of the skin of the breast. Superficial phlebitis is self-limiting, the pain subsiding within a few weeks.

3 In pregnancy this is a physiological change and does not signify any underlying malignancy, nor has it the sinister links with malignancy that superficial phlebitis carries at other sites, e.g. thrombophlebitis migrans. However, if the condition arises outside pregnancy, it may be a manifestation of underlying malignancy.

## B

1 Raynaud's phenomenon.

2 Small vessel diseases, e.g. vasculitis, vasospastic disorders, large vessel disease and Raynaud's disease where there are no precipitating or predisposing conditions.

3 In response to a fall in temperature, normal arterioles and capillaries close down and blood is diverted from the capillary bed by arteriovenous shunts. In Raynaud's syndrome the response to a change of temperature is accentuated, influenced by the autonomic system and emotion. The affected part turns white initially as the temperature falls. As re-warming occurs, it turns first blue and then red, from a reactive hyperaemia, which is often very painful.

## C

1 Figure (a) shows a fracture blister in a patient with a fracture of the right calcaneum. Figure (b) shows a haematoma associated with a facial injury.

2 Skin, vascular, muscular, nerve and visceral injury.

3 An untreated fracture three to five days after injury, most commonly seen around the lower leg.

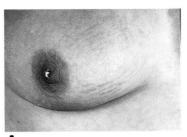

**A**

1  What does this figure show?

2  What are the causes of this disorder?

3  What other types of nipple discharge are there?

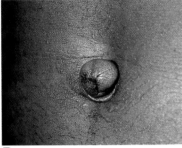

**B**

1  What is the diagnosis?

2  List other abnormalities of the umbilicus.

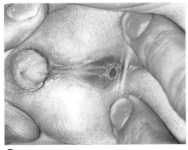

**C**

1  What is the diagnosis?

2  What other abnormalities occur in this condition?

3  What is the treatment?

# Answers page 121

## A

1 Nipple discharge in a patient with galactorrhoea.

2 Galactorrhoea may be physiological, i.e. lactation during or after pregnancy, or pathological. Pathological causes include: hyperprolactinaemia resulting from a prolactinoma, polycystic ovaries, liver failure or may be idiopathic. It may also be secondary to drug therapy, e.g. oestrogens, opiates, cimetidine, dopamine antagonists.

3 (a) Bloodstained – benign duct papilloma, ductal carcinoma, rarely carcinoma in a lactating breast
  (b) slightly bloodstained fluid – together with the presence of a cystic swelling of the breast is strongly suggestive of an intracystic papillary carcinoma
  (c) clear or yellow serous fluid – benign breast disease, secondary to the oral contraceptive pill
  (d) thick green discharge – duct ectasia owing to hyperproliferative duct tissue producing a cellular discharge.

## B

1 Umbilical fibroma.

2 ● Congenital – exomphalos; patent urachus or vitellointestinal duct; hernia
  ● paraumbilical hernias
  ● inflammation – omphalitis; granuloma; dermatitis; concretion, pilonidal sinus
  ● neoplasia – benign adenoma; endometriosis; malignant: primary extension of intra-abdominal pathology; secondary (Sister Joseph's nodule)
  ● venous dilatation.

## C

1 Perineal hypospadias, which accounts for 15 per cent of cases of hypospadias.

2 Cordi of the penis, which is ventral angulation caused by the presence of fibrous tissue within the penile fascia. Undescended testis and inguinal hernias also occur.

3 If it is a glandular defect a glandular meatotomy is performed. However, more severe cases require urethroplasty and meatal advancement.

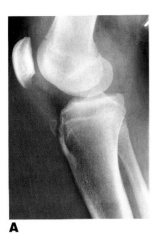

**A**

1  What is the diagnosis?
2  Which age group is most affected by this condition?
3  What pathological processes are involved in this disease?

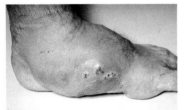

**B**

1  What is the diagnosis of this lesion in a barefoot youth in Central America?
2  What is the causative organism?
3  What is the initial manifestation of this lesion?

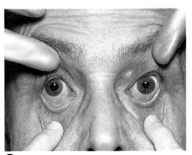

**C**

1  What are the causes of yellow discoloration of the sclera?
2  How would you assess this sign?

# Answers page 123

## A

1  Osgood–Schlatter's disease.

2  It occurs in adolescents during their growth spurt and is common in athletic youngsters.

3  (a) Avascular necrosis
   (b)     traction injury
   (c) fracture or separation of the fragments.

## B

1  Madura foot.

2  Fungal infection.

3  The infection first manifests as a firm, painless, rather pale nodule, usually on the foot. The lesion later increases in size and others appear. Vesicles occur in about a week, followed by discharge and sinus formation.

## C

1  Causes of jaundice:
   - haemolytic (prehepatic) disorders – hereditary spherocytosis; hypersplenism
   - liver (hepatic) dysfunction – hepatitis, cirrhosis; metabolic disorders
   - obstructed biliary tree – intraluminal (gallstones); in the wall (benign, malignant strictures, sclerosing cholangitis); outside the wall (pancreatic, hepatic tumours).

2  - History: colour of urine, stool, infection, diseases, travel, work, drugs and hepatotoxins
   - investigations: LFT, abdominal US or CT, ERCP
   - physical examination: hyperdynamic circulation, bounding pulse, body hair loss, spider naevi – more than nine new crops indicates progressive disease, palmar erythema, particularly the thenar and hypothenar eminences, liver palms, Dupuytren's contracture, leukonychia and clubbing, liver flap, hepatomegaly, ascites, mental changes.

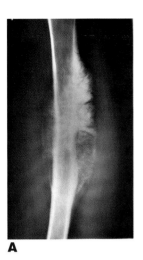

**A**

1  Describe this radiograph.
2  What is the diagnosis?
3  Which age groups are most affected?

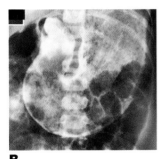

**B**

A 12-year-old, anxious girl presented with epigastric distension and excessive vomiting, with the radiological features shown.

1  What is this phenomenon called?
2  What are the complications?

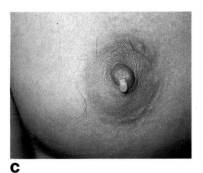

**C**

1  What is the diagnosis?
2  What is the common cause?
3  What are common causes of discharge from the nipple?

# Answers page 125

### A

1  Swelling of the middle of the left femur, with both destruction and new bone formation. The periosteal bone invades the muscles, the bone has a sun-ray appearance and Codman's triangle is present at the junction of the cortex with the periosteum.

2  Osteosarcoma of the bone.

3  Seventy-five per cent of patients are between the ages of 10 and 25 years. In the elderly it is a complication of Paget's disease of the bone.

### B

1  Trichobezoar – if the ingested material is hair.

2  Mucosal ulceration; perforation by sharp objects; moulding into a mass; pyloric obstruction.

### C

1  Galactorrhoea.

2  Prolactinoma.

3  ● Fresh blood – duct papilloma, carcinoma
   ● altered blood – duct papilloma, carcinoma
   ● bloodstained – carcinoma
   ● serous (clear, yellow, green) – benign breast disease
   ● thick (brown, green) – duct ectasia
   ● milky – lactation, galactorrhoea.

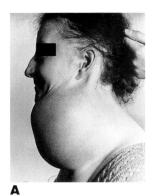

**A**

1   What is this lesion?
2   How is this condition produced?
3   What are the symptoms?

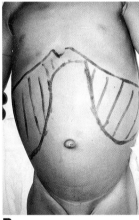

**B**

The figure shows massive hepatosplenomegaly.

1   If it is tender, give three bacterial and three viral causes.

2   If it is non-tender give three bacterial and three protozoal or parasitic causes.

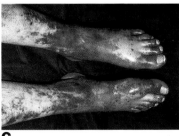

**C**

1   What does DIC stand for?
2   What clinical conditions can cause it?
3   What is the pathophysiology of this condition?

# Answers page 127

## A

1  Extensive multinodular goitre.

2  A disordered thyroid metabolism, where some areas of the gland become hyperplastic and form nodules which later degenerate, fibrose and calcify.

3  Symptoms of a swelling in the neck (dyspnoea, hoarseness, dysphagia) and those related to the endocrine activity of the gland.

## B

1  Brucellosis, typhoid fever, borreliosis, bartonellosis; Epstein–Barr virus, viral hepatitis, cytomegalovirus.

2  Tuberculosis, leprosy, syphilis, schistosomiasis, kala-azar, hydatid liver disease.

## C

1  Disseminated intravascular coagulation.

2  DIC can be associated with malignancy (adenocarcinoma of the gut, prostate, ovary and leukaemia), Gram-negative septicaemia, fat embolism, trauma and amniotic fluid embolism.

3  DIC is a consumption coagulopathy, which causes laying down of fibrin throughout the micro-circulation. This is followed by fibrinolysis, depletion of clotting factors and thrombocytopenia. The patient therefore presents with widespread haemorrhage.

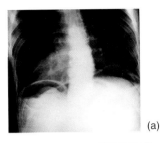

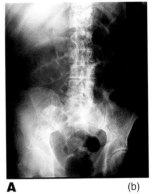

(a)

**A**                    (b)

1   What is the most likely diagnosis in this patient with a three-hour history of acute abdominal pain?

2   What is meant by right paracolic gutter phenomenon?

3   What are the most important physical signs in judging the seriousness of this problem?

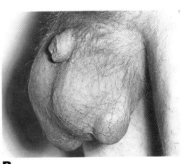

**B**

1   What does this figure demonstrate?

2   What are the differences between direct and indirect inguinal herniae?

3   What causes intestinal obstruction in these lesions?

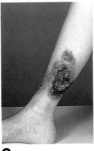

**C**

1   This patient has an ulcer secondary to inflammatory bowel disease. What is the lesion called?

2   What other extraintestinal manifestations of inflammatory bowel disease may occur?

3   What medical treatment options are available in the management of inflammatory bowel disease?

# Answers page 129

## A

1  Perforated peptic ulcer: figure (a) air under the diaphragm, figure (b) air between loops of gut.

2  It is a diagnostic pitfall; this occurs after a duodenal perforation. The leaking duodenal fluid is directed downwards alongside the ascending colon into the right iliac fossa and the signs can be confused with appendicitis.

3  The general condition of the patient, in particular the pulse and blood pressure, are the most important factors. A pulse rate of more than 100 is associated with a grave prognosis.

## B

1  Left indirect inguinal hernia, with the testis sited inferoposteriorly. It is possible to get above the scrotal swelling on the right, which is a collection of spermatoceles.

2  Direct herniae rarely descend into the scrotum, are revealed more easily when the patient lies down and emerge directly forward, rather than obliquely. They appear later in life and are rare in women. They do not occur in children and rarely strangulate.

3  The narrow neck of the sac is the main factor in producing hernial obstruction.

## C

1  Pyoderma gangrenosum.

2  Some manifestations are related to disease activity. These include: on the skin – pyoderma and erythema nodosum; mucous membranes may develop aphthous ulcers. Patients may also have iritis and arthritis of large joints. Some manifestations are unrelated to disease activity. Joints may develop a sacroiliitis and ankylosing spondylitis. Chronic active hepatitis and cirrhosis of the liver may occur and sclerosing cholangitis and bile duct carcinoma are associated. Crohn's disease has an increased incidence of renal amyloidosis and finger clubbing may occur.

3  Anti-inflammatory agents are used. Steroids can be used to produce a remission and sulphasalazine to maintain remissions, although it may need to be taken for at least a year. Symptomatic control for diarrhoea – codeine phosphate or loperamide. Nutritional supplements may be required if the patient is unwell or malnourished. This can be oral or intravenous. In chronic, cases patients often need iron supplementation.

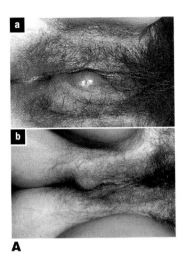

**A**

1  What is the most likely diagnosis of figures (a) and (b)?

2  What are the differential diagnoses?

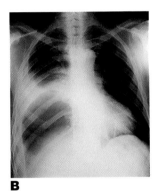

**B**

1  What does this radiograph show?

2  What are the commonest causes of this condition?

3  How may this patient present?

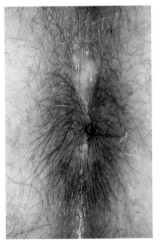

**C**

1  Describe this figure of a patient with an insatiable itch around the anal region.

2  What are the common causes of pruritus ani?

# Answers page 131

## A

1  (a) Bartholin abscess;
(b) Bartholin cyst.

2  Sebaceous cyst, subcutaneous benign or malignant tumours, lipomas, fibromas, neurofibromas, leiomyomas and vascular lesions.

## B

1  Large subphrenic abscess with a highly displaced right dome of the diaphragm.

2  Perforated peptic ulcer, abdominal trauma, perforation of the biliary tree, stomach, large bowel or appendix. The perforation may be an inflammatory or malignant lesion or may be iatrogenic, e.g. following instrumentation or surgery.

3  The patient usually looks unwell, with anorexia, nausea and tachycardia. Upper abdominal or back pain is usual which may radiate to the shoulder. Occasionally hiccups are present owing to diaphragmatic irritation. There is a swinging pyrexia and occasionally rigors.

## C

1  Erythematous discoloration around the anal orifice resulting from itching and scratching.

2  Pruritus ani:
- generalized itch – obstructive jaundice; diabetes mellitus; hyperparathyroidism; myeloproliferative disorders; lymphoma
- local factors – excess sweating; poor hygiene; woollen underwear
- skin conditions – eczema; allergy; contact dermatitis; lichen planus; psoriasis
- infections/infestations – sexually transmitted diseases; fungal; scabies; lice; threadworms
- diarrhoea/incontinence – leakage of liquid paraffin; sphincter malfunction; rectal prolapse
- anal pathology – piles; fissures; fistulae; warts; Crohn's disease; TB; polyps; cancer
- rectal pathology – solitary ulcer; benign and malignant tumours
- in women – candidiasis; trichomoniasis; urinary leakage
- psychological causes
- nappy rash.

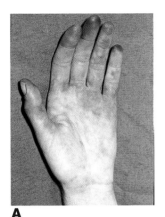

A

1   What is the diagnosis?

2   What may cause this condition?

3   What are the clinical features of this condition?

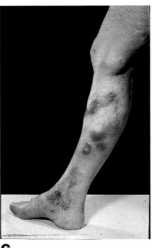

B

1   What condition is present in this young man?

2   What is the pathophysiology of this condition?

3   What are the causes?

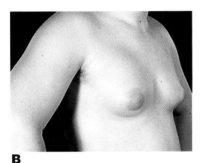

C

1   What is the diagnosis?

2   What is the resting venous pressure at calf level when standing and what mechansim returns venous blood to the heart?

3   Does the blood drain from the superficial to the deep venous system and, if so, why?

# Answers page 133

## A

1  Acute ischaemia to the left hand.

2  Embolus, vasospasm following cannulation or intra-arterial drug injection, AV fistula formation.

3  Pain, pallor, pulseless, paralysis, perishingly cold and paraesthesia (the six Ps).

## B

1  Bilateral gynaecomastia.

2  It is produced in response to elevated levels of oestrogen or oestrogen-like compounds.

3  ● Physiological – neonatal owing to circulating maternal hormones; puberty usually recovering spontaneously; old age
   ● hypogonadism – gonadotrophin insufficiency; decreased Leydig cell function; androgen resistance
   ● tumours – testicular, adrenal and those producing ectopic hormones, such as bronchogenic carcinoma
   ● hepatic – reduced oestrogen breakdown
   ● hyperthyroidism – increased sex hormone binding globulin and increased sex hormone production
   ● iatrogenic – oestrogen therapy, cimetidine, neurotransmitter agonists, spironolactone, digitalis.

## C

1  Thrombosis of the long saphenous vein.

2  Resting venous pressure is 100–130 cm $H_2O$. When the calf muscles contract a pressure of 100 mm Hg[1] is produced, which compresses the deep veins in the calf and propels blood towards the heart. The effectiveness of this muscle pump is dependent on the venous valves being intact.

3  Yes. The contraction of calf muscles forces blood proximally out of the deep veins towards the heart, reducing pressure within the deep system. This produces a pressure gradient and blood flows from the superficial to the deep veins: the valves prevent reverse flow.

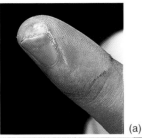
(a)

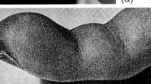
(b)

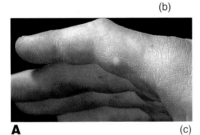

**A** (c)

1   What are the diagnoses of these lesions?

2   What anatomical sites would you expect to be involved?

3   What are the principles of treatment?

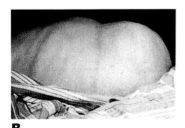

**B**

1   What is the abnormality in this patient?

2   What are the differential diagnoses?

3   What are the causes of acute urinary retention?

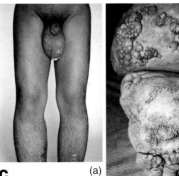

**C** (a)

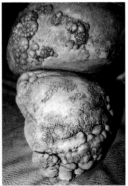

(b)

1   Describe these figures.

2   What is the most likely causative agent?

3   What is another term for this disease?

# Answers page 135

## A

1   Hand infections:
   - Figure (a) – apical abscess
   - Figure (b) – pulp space infection
   - Figure (c) – septic arthritis following pulp space infection.

2   - Apical – lies beneath the free edge of the nail, following a penetrating injury such as a splinter
   - pulp space – on the palmar aspect, in the subcutaneous fat.

3   Evacuation of pus, appropriate antibiotic therapy followed by rest and elevation.

## B

1   There is a large abdominal mass arising from the pelvis and extending above the umbilicus.

2   Distended bladder, pregnant uterus, fibroid, ovarian cyst, bladder tumour, other pelvic malignancy.

3   Enlarged prostate, either owing to benign prostatic hypertrophy or adenocarcinoma. Urethral stricture, urethral or bladder stone, prostate chips obstructing the bladder neck following transurethral resection of the prostate, foreign body, transitional cell carcinoma at the bladder neck causing obstruction, urinary tract infection in men, neuropathic bladder, post spinal injury.

## C

1   Figure (a): secondary lymphoedema of the legs and scrotum from filarial infection; figure (b): severe secondary lymphoedema of the lower leg owing to filarial infection.

2   *Wuncheria bancrofti*, which is a roundworm.

3   Elephantiasis.

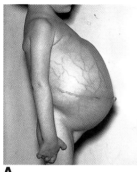

**A**

1   What does this figure show?
2   What are the possible causes of this?

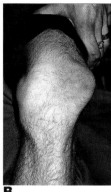

(a)

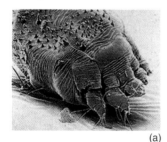

**B**

1   What does this figure show?
2   How does this condition present?
3   What are the predisposing factors?

**C**                              (b)

1   What do figures (a) and (b) show?
2   Into what group do these organisms fall?
3   What effects do these parasites produce?

# Answers page 137

## A

1 Abdominal distension in a child.

2 Intestinal obstruction, distended bladder secondary to urethral obstruction, congenital cystic kidneys, neonatal ascites, meconium peritonitis.

## B

1 Lateral dislocation of the patella.

2 Following a direct blow or without injury if there is a predisposing factor, the knee is locked in flexion with a haemarthrosis. Not infrequently an osteochondral fragment is sheared off during dislocation and diagnosed by radiograph. Examine the lateral radiograph for evidence of a lipohaemarthrosis, i.e. fat floating on top of the effusion in the suprapatellar bursa. If in doubt, aspirate for fat globules.

3 Predisposing factors are a high patella, a low lateral femoral condyle, a small patella and marked knock knees.

## C

1 Figure (a) shows the itch mite *Sarcoptes scabiei*; figure (b) shows the wound produced when the female burrows into the skin to lay her eggs, producing intense itching, usually on the dorsum of the web space.

2 Jointed arthropods.

3 Their bites may be painful and cause hypersensitivity and itching. They may also carry diseases, particularly epidemic typhus and relapsing fever.

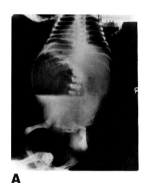

**A**

1 What is the most likely diagnosis in this 10-day-old infant with abdominal distension and a failure to pass meconium since birth?

2 What are the other causes of abdominal distension?

3 What would you expect to find on rectal examination?

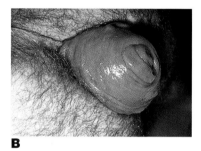

**B**

1 What is the diagnosis?

2 How would you differentiate it from prolapse of rectal mucosa?

3 What are the predisposing factors?

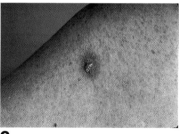

**C**

1 Describe this lesion.

2 What is the most likely diagnosis?

3 How is the lesion produced?

# Answers page 139

## A

1  Meconium peritonitis.

2  Intestinal obstruction, distended bladder secondary to urethral obstruction, congenital cystic kidneys, neonatal ascites.

3  PR reveals a narrow rectum and anus and, after the finger is withdrawn, only rarely does the normal passage of meconium result.

## B

1  Prolapse of the rectum.

2  The two can be distinguished by feeling one wall of the prolapse between the index finger and thumb. A full-thickness prolapse feels like a double-layered tube.

3  Extremes of age (elderly and childhood), children with chronic malnutrition or chronic diarrhoea.

## C

1  Red induration with central debris.

2  Foreign body granuloma.

3  Subcutaneous implantation of external debris and bacteria.

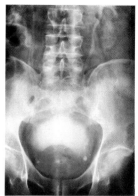
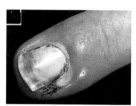

**A**

1   What is the abnormality in this radiograph?

2   What are the differential diagnoses?

3   Which part of the prostate enlarges in benign prostatic hypertrophy?

**B**

1   What is the diagnosis?

2   What is the most common causative organism?

3   How would you explain the site of the infection?

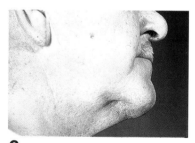

**C**

1   What is the most likely diagnosis in this patient with a past history of a tooth abscess?

2   What is the cause of the associated bluish-green purulent discharge?

3   How would you treat the condition?

# Answers page 141

## A

1  There is a filling defect in the base of the bladder.

2  Enlarged prostate, or bladder tumour.

3  The central zone usually enlarges and bulges into the prostatic urethra, hence causing obstruction to urinary flow and producing the typical obstructive and irritative symptoms of prostatism.

## B

1  Acute paronychia.

2  Staphylococcal infection.

3  Initially infection arises underneath a torn nail or damaged cuticle and spreads around the nail. In 60 per cent of cases pus extends underneath the nail (subungual abscess).

## C

1  Sinus from a tooth abscess.

2  Bluish-green pus is characteristic of *Pseudomonas* infection.

3  A chronic abscess and sterile collections resolve only after adequate drainage and debridement. It will not resolve if foreign bodies such as prostheses, mesh, bone sequestra, necrotic tendon or an infected root remain.

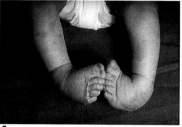

**A**

1 What is the diagnosis?
2 What is the incidence of this abnormality?
3 What are the predisposing factors?

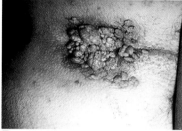

**B**

1 What is the diagnosis?
2 What is the causative agent?
3 Which group of people is most affected?
4 What is the clinical presentation?

**C**

1 What does this figure show?
2 What are the signs of liver failure?
3 What are the causes of clubbing?

# Answers page 143

## A

1 Talipes equinovarus.

2 Approximately 1:1000 live births.

3 A strong familial tendency, boys are affected twice as often as girls, increased uterine pressure may also predispose (uterine packaging).

## B

1 Perianal warts (condylomata accuminata).

2 Human papillomavirus.

3 The highest incidence is in homosexual males, the condition being almost invariably sexually transmitted.

4 The patient usually complains of itching, bleeding and perianal lumps

## C

1 Signs of chronic liver disease, i.e. spider naevi, palmar erythema and clubbing.

2 Other signs of liver failure include a bounding pulse, body hair loss, leukonychia and Dupuytren's contracture. Later signs include jaundice, gynaecomastia, testicular atrophy, ascites, liver flap, hepatic encephalopathy, convulsions and coma.

3 (a) Cardiovascular: congenital cyanotic heart disease, subacute bacterial endocarditis
(b) respiratory: fibrosing alveolitis, chronic suppurative lung disease, e.g. bronchiectasis, bronchial carcinoma, pleural and mediastinal tumours
(c) GI: cirrhosis, liver failure, inflammatory bowel disease
(d) idiopathic/congenital.

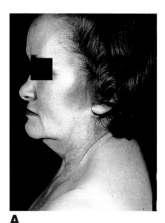

**A**

1  What is the diagnosis?

2  What is the pathology of this disease?

3  What investigations would confirm the diagnosis?

4  What are the clinical features of this disease?

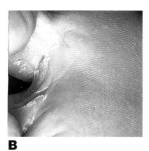

**B**

1  Describe the lesion shown.

2  What is the likely diagnosis?

3  What is the causative agent?

4  Where would you expect to find such a lesion?

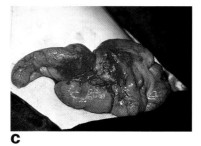

**C**

1  What does this figure show?

2  What is the classical manifestation of this disease?

3  What are the principles behind the treatment of this disease?

# Answers page 145

## A

1  Paget's disease.

2  Paget's disease is a bony disorder of unknown aetiology. There is greatly increased bone turnover, with excessive osteoclastic resorption, although there is equivalent osteoblastic activity to replace bone. The bone formed is soft and lacks normal mineralization.

3  (a) Very high levels of serum alkaline phosphatase owing to excess bone turnover (may be greater than 1000 IU $l^{-1}$)
   (b) a mixture of osteolytic and osteosclerotic lesions demonstrated radiologically
   (c) isotope bone scanning identifies affected bones but does not differentiate Paget's disease from other disorders, e.g. metastatic disease.

4  The major symptom is usually localized bone pain, which may be severe and continuous. Pathological fractures may occur owing to the replaced bone being fragile and brittle. Overgrowth of any bone can occur but common sites affected are the skull (causing frontal bossing and compression of cranial nerves) and long bones (causing bowing of the bone). In 1 per cent of patients there is sarcomatous malignant change.

## B

1  Maceration between the toes.

2  Tinea pedis.

3  Fungal infection.

4  It is usually found in the web and interspace of the toes involved but may infect the nail fold and produce chronic paronychia and a ridged, brown pigmented nail.

## C

1  An operative photograph of an acute appendicitis.

2  The classical history is of gradual onset of central colicky abdominal pain over twenty-four hours, associated with anorexia, nausea and occasionally vomiting. The pain shifts to the right iliac fossa and the pain is aggravated by vomiting or coughing.

3  As the photograph shows, the cause is acute appendicitis and the appendix must be removed.

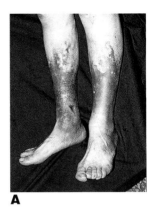

**A**

1   What skin changes have occurred with this ulcer?

2   What are the characteristics of a venous versus an arterial ulcer?

3   What is a Marjolin's ulcer?

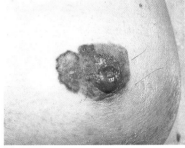

**B**

1   What are the skin changes shown?

2   What is the diagnosis?

3   How does this condition differ from eczematous changes resulting from dermatitis?

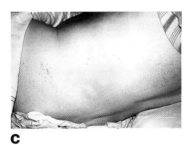

**C**

1   What is the name of this sign?

2   What is the associated disease?

3   What other sign may be present?

4   What else may cause flank discoloration?

# Answers page 147

## A

1  Hyperpigmentation, swelling and induration. These together are known as lipodermatosclerosis.

2  Venous ulcers are sited above the ankle, have gently sloping edges, with granulation tissue at the base, peripheral pulses are present. There may be varicose veins and lipodermatosclerosis and the limb is usually warm. Arterial ulcers are sited on or between the toes or on pressure sites, such as the heel, metacarpophalangeal joints and the malleoli, tend to have a punched-out appearance and do not heal well. There are diminished or absent peripheral pulses and cyanosis and rubor of the skin. There may be slough within the ulcer and the limb is usually cold.

3  This is malignant change which occurs at the periphery of a long-standing venous ulcer. It is usually a squamous cell carcinoma.

## B

1  Eczema of the nipple or Paget's disease.

2  Paget's disease with underlying neoplastic spread through the duct system.

3  Initially the appearances are similar, but Paget's disease is unilateral and slowly erodes and completely destroys the nipple.

## C

1  Grey Turner's sign.

2  Severe haemorrhagic pancreatitis.

3  Cullen's sign (discoloration around the umbilicus).

4  Any cause of retroperitoneal bleeding (usually leakage from an abdominal aortic or iliac artery aneurysm).

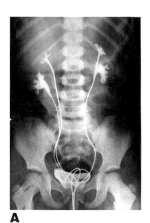

**A**

1  What is this investigation and what does it show?
2  How do the ureters enter the bladder?
3  How may this condition present?

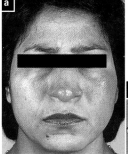
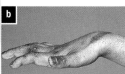

**B**

1  Describe these lesions.
2  What is the diagnosis?
3  What sites are commonly involved?

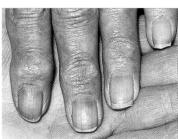
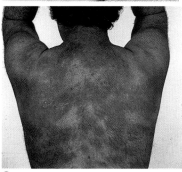

**C**

1  What is this disease?
2  Where is the pigmentation commonly sited?
3  What is the pathophysiology of the pigmentation?

# Answers page 149

## A

1  Retrograde pyelogram. It shows a right duplex collecting system.

2  The upper moiety ureter enters the bladder below the lower pole ureter and more medially.

3  It is usually asymptomatic and is found incidentally on intravenous urogram (IVU) or at cystoscopy. These patients have an increased incidence of urinary tract infections and ureteric reflux. There may be urinary leakage if the lower ureter opens below the external urethral sphincter.

## B

1  Figure (a): cutaneous facial lesion, with thickening of the nerve; figure (b): muscle wasting of the hand.

2  Leprosy.

3  Superficial portion of the peripheral nerves, e.g. the ulnar nerve above the elbow, the greater auricular nerve in the neck and the radial and median nerves at the wrist.

## C

1  Addison's disease.

2  Pigmentation is commonly in skin creases, e.g. palms, scars, lips and cheeks and on exposed areas such as the back.

3  There is decreased circulation of cortisol owing to adrenal failure and a reduced negative feedback to the pituitary gland increases serum ACTH. Since ACTH has a melanocyte simulating hormone activity, there is increased melanin production and, therefore, pigmentation.

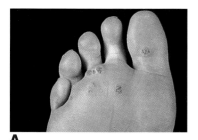

1  What is this lesion?
2  What is the causative organism?
3  What site(s) are commonly involved?

**A**

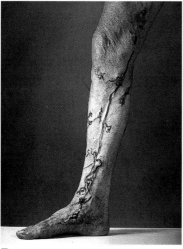

1  What clinical tests would you perform to confirm incompetence of venous valves in varicose vein disease?
2  What are the tributaries at the saphenovarix?
3  What treatment options are available for a person with varicose veins?

**B**

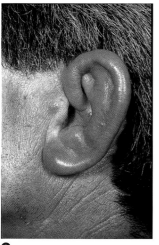

1  How would you define this lesion?
2  How would you differentiate it from cellulitis?
3  What is the main site and point of entry?
4  What is meant by Milian's ear sign?

**C**

# Answers page 151

### A

1  Plantar wart.

2  The wart is produced by infection with the human papillomavirus.

3  Plantar warts occur on the weight-bearing areas of the ball of the foot or heel.

### B

1  Cough impulse test, where the fingers are placed over the saphenovarix and the patient is asked to cough. The percussion test, where saphenous or lower segments are tapped to assess which valves are incompetent. Brodie–Trendelenburg test for assessing competence of the saphenofemoral junction or the perforating veins. Perthes' test for deep venous competence.

2  The long saphenous vein, superficial inferior epigastric vein, superficial circumflex iliac vein, superficial external pudendal vein and the medial superficial circumflex iliac vein.

3  Conservative treatment comprises elasticated stockings. Surgical management is by ligation of the saphenofemoral or the saphenopopliteal junction with vein stripping and avulsion of tributaries. Injection sclerotherapy, using sodium tetradecyl 1 per cent, is followed by three weeks' compression bandaging.

### C

1  Erysipelas – streptococcal cellulitis of the skin and subcutaneous tissue.

2  Erysipelas is caused by streptococci and cellulitis is caused mainly by staphylococci, which cause localized infection and pus formation. Streptococcus spreads easily, causing oedema of the involved skin and giving the area a raised border of infection.

3  The face is the most common site; oedema is prominent and may completely close the eyelids. The point of entry is usually obscure, although careful examination may reveal a source of entry such as a small cut or a scratch.

4  This sign differentiates non-specific cellulitis from erysipelas in that the latter involves the pinna because it is a cuticular lymphangitis. Subcutaneous inflammation stops short of the pinna because of the close adherence of the skin to the cartilage.

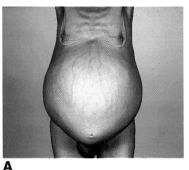

**A**

1   What does this figure show?

2   What are the possible causes of this condition?

3   What physical signs would you expect to find in this patient?

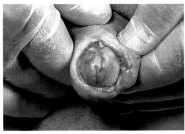

**B**

1   What is the diagnosis?

2   What pre-malignant conditions may exist on the penis?

3   What treatment options are available?

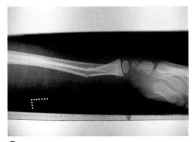

**C**

1   Describe this fracture.

2   Which age group is most likely to be affected?

3   What other types of fracture affect this age group?

# Answers page 153

## A

1  Gross ascites

2  (a) Straw-coloured ascites – malignancy, cirrhosis, infective (TB or following intra-abdominal perforation), hypoproteinaemia (e.g. in nephrotic syndrome), constrictive pericarditis, hepatic vein obstruction (e.g. Budd–Chiari syndrome, chronic pancreatitis, Meig's syndrome).
(b) chylous ascites – obstruction of main lymphatic ducts.
(c) haemorrhagic ascites – malignancy, ruptured ectopic pregnancy, abdominal trauma, acute pancreatitis.

3  Fluid thrill, shifting dullness.

## B

1  Invasive squamous cell carcinoma of the penis.

2  Leukoplakia, erythroplasia of Queyrat (this is carcinoma in situ), cutaneous horn, which is an overgrowth and cornification of the epithelium.

3  Small, localized lesions can be treated with external beam radiotherapy. Enlarged lymph nodes should be treated initially with antibiotics and, if still present at six weeks, should be biopsied. If tumour is present then inguinal block dissection is performed. More advanced lesions are treated by partial or radical penile amputation. The presence of fixed lymph nodes requires palliative radiotherapy, while metastatic disease can be treated with chemotherapy.

## C

1  Greenstick fracture of the left radius. It is an incomplete fracture leaving cortex and periosteum intact on one side of the bone.

2  It most commonly affects children.

3  Other fractures particularly affecting children include: (i) plastic deformation with angulation as a result of binding; (ii) fractures involving the epiphysis.

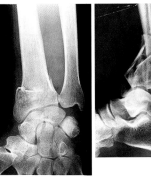

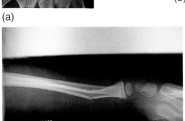

(a)

(b)

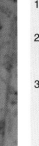

**A**

(c)

1   What do these figures show?

2   What types of displacement do they show?

3   What are the clinical findings?

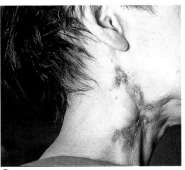

**B**

1   What are the differential diagnoses of this swelling?

2   On surgical exploration caseous material was evacuated: what is the likely diagnosis?

3   Where is the most common site of entry of this organism?

**C**

1   Describe this figure.

2   What are the stages of this disease?

# Answers page 155

## A

1 Figure (a) impacted fracture, (b) comminuted fracture and (c) greenstick fracture.

2 Displacement, a shift of alignment, angulation, shortening, twist and distraction.

3 Local pain, tenderness, swelling, loss of function, deformity and crepitus.

## B

1 Parotid abscess, periauricular tuberculosis, parotid malignancy.

2 Tuberculous abscess: surgery is indicated when there is no local response to chemotherapy and if a sinus is formed.

3 In most cases, tubercle bacilli gain entrance through the tonsil of the corresponding side.

## C

1 Chronic scarring following chronic inflammation (tuberculosis).

2 Stage I – enlarged firm nodes.
Stage II – local abscess.
Stage III – spreading pus – collar stud abscess.
Stage IV – spontaneous or surgical discharge with sinus formation.

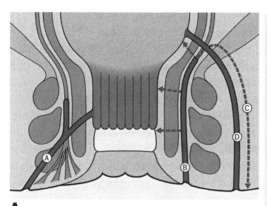

**A**

1  What do the letters A, B, C and D represent?

2  How may these patients present?

3  What is Goodsall's rule?

4  What is a seton?

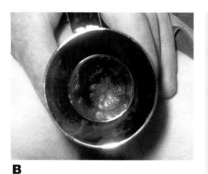

**B**

1  What does this figure show?

2  What are the commonest types of tumour found in this region?

3  How do these tumours present?

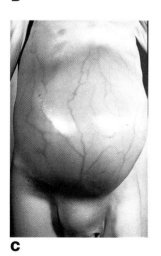

**C**

1  What is the cause of the hernia in this figure?

2  How do you approach the treatment of this hernia?

3  What are the contraindications for surgical intervention?

# Answers page 157

### A

1   The four main types of anal fistula (according to Parks' classification):
    A   trans-sphincteric (high or low)
    B   intersphincteric
    C   suprasphincteric
    D   extrasphincteric (supralevator).

2   Patients with anal fistulae complain of intermittent anal pain and discharge (either purulent or mixed with blood). There is often a history of acute anal sepsis which has either settled after spontaneous discharge of pus or has needed surgical intervention.

3   Goodsall's rule states that for openings anterior to a transverse mid-anal line, the fistula runs radially into the anal canal. For openings posterior to this line, the track opens in the posterior midline of the anal canal.

4   These are ligatures (usually made from nylon) which are used in the treatment of high or complicated fistulae. They are placed through the track of a fistula and may be applied loosely (when used as a drain) or tightly to stimulate fibrosis. The fibrosis prevents separation of the anal sphincter muscle when gradual fistulotomy (by regular tightening of the seton) is performed.

### B

1   Melanoma of the anal canal.

2   Anal carcinomas are most commonly squamous cell carcinomas, whereas low rectal carcinomas tend to be adenocarcinomas.

3   Anal tumours present as either painful or painless lumps in the anus, usually with bleeding. Anal squamous cell carcinomas appear warty, as an indurated plaque or as an ulcer. Melanomas are usually wart-like pigmented tumours. Spread from anal tumours is usually to the inguinal lymph nodes. Rectal tumours usually present with change in bowel habit, rectal bleeding or tenesmus. These tumours spread to pelvic lymph nodes and to the liver.

### C

1   Increase in intra-abdominal pressure due to ascites.

2   Treatment of ascites, i.e. the precipitating factor must be treated before hernial repair.

3   If the general condition of the patient is poor, e.g. in a patient with chronic cough, bladder neck obstruction or ascites, one should avoid interfering with the hernia. In large, long-standing herniae (e.g. fifteen years) reduction and repair may lead to respiratory embarrassment and is another contraindication to surgical intervention. In ascitic patients, surgery leads to the escape of ascitic fluid through the wound.

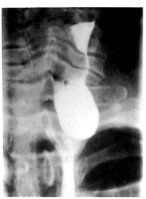

**A**

1   What is the diagnosis?

2   Where in the pharynx is it most likely to occur?

3   What are the presenting features?

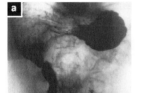

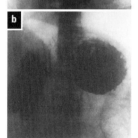

**B**

1   What do these radiographs show?

2   What is the mechanism of these lesions?

3   What are the manifestations of this condition?

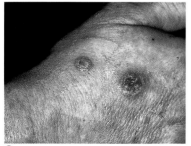

**C**

1   What is the diagnosis of this lesion in a 35-year-old farmer?

2   What is the causative organism?

3   What is the source of infection?

# Answers page 159

## A

1  This is a pharyngeal pouch.

2  These commonly occur at Killian's dehiscence, i.e. between the thyropharyngeal and cricopharyngeal muscles. This is the weakest point in the pharyngeal wall.

3  The patient complains of dysphagia, regurgitation of undigested food and weight loss. Less frequently patients may complain of a hoarse voice and recurrent chest infections caused by overspill into the lungs.

## B

1  Volvulus of the stomach: (a) organoaxial, (b) mesenterioaxial.

2  As the stomach is fixed at the lower end of the oesophagus and the first part of the duodenum, occasionally the organ can rotate between these points, either along its axis (organoaxial) or at right angles to this plane (mesenterioaxial).

3  Fullness, vomiting, retching, abdominal pain. A stomach tube cannot be passed.

## C

1  Orf infection.

2  Poxvirus.

3  Animal contact – the virus is carried by sheep, cattle and goats.

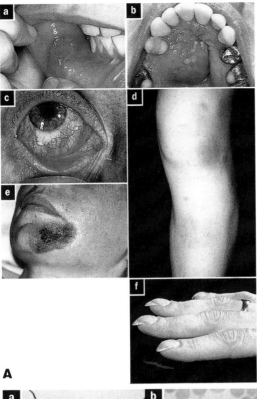

**A**

1 What are these extra-intestinal manifestations of chronic inflammatory bowel disease?

2 What other extra-intestinal lesions occur?

3 How do you differentiate between different types of inflammatory bowel disease?

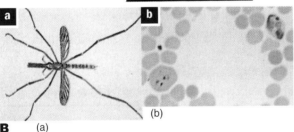

**B**  (a)  (b)

1 Describe these figures.

2 What is the mode of transmission?

3 What is the common presentation of this lesion?

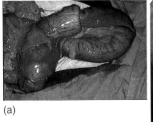

(a)  (b)

**C**

1 What do these figures show?

2 What is the process by which this condition may cause obstruction?

3 What are the common causes of this condition?

4 How may this condition present in infants?

# Answers page 161

## A

1  a, Crohn's lesion of lip; b, palatal Crohn's; c, episcleritis; d, erythema nodosum; f, clubbing.

2  Aphthous ulcers, iridocyclitis, arthritis, biliary cirrhosis, pericholangitis, cholelithiasis, drug reactions, nephritis.

3

| | Ulcerative colitis | Crohn's disease |
| --- | --- | --- |
| Usual location | Rectum, left colon | Anywhere |
| Rectal involvement and bleeding | Almost always | Uncommon |
| Fistula | Rare | Common |
| Stricture | Rare | Common |

## B

1  (a) Female *Anopheles mosquito*: the transmitter of malaria; (b) intracellular *Plasmodium falciparum* in a blood film.

2  Blood-sucking female *Anopheles* mosquito.

3  Fever (the timing of rigors is often diagnostic) with intense shivering. The importance to the surgeon is mainly in the differential diagnosis of fever, anaemia, abdominal pain, jaundice, diarrhoea and hepatosplenomegaly.

## C

1  (a) Small bowel intussusception; (b) barium study showing colocolonic intussusception.

2  An intussusception is the invagination of a segment of bowel into an adjacent loop. The mesentery is drawn in between the two loops and the blood supply may thus be compromised, leading to strangulation and perforation. The cause of an intussusception is usually a lesion at the apex of the inverted loop, which is drawn distally by peristalsis of the outer loop.

3  Most commonly this is due to an enlarged Peyer's patch, e.g. in response to viral or bacterial infection of the gut. The causative lesion may also be benign, e.g. a polyp, or malignant, e.g. colonic carcinoma, or may be due to a gut abnormality, e.g. Meckel's diverticulum.

4  It is commoner in male infants (usually aged 6–24 months) and presents with a sudden onset of colicky abdominal pain. The pain may cause drawing up of the legs and screaming attacks. The pain becomes more severe and prolonged as the disease progresses. Vomiting and distension appear. The diagnostic feature is the presence of a redcurrant jelly-like stool.

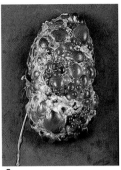

**A**

1  What is the diagnosis?

2  What is the mode of inheritance and what is the age of presentation?

3  How is this condition managed?

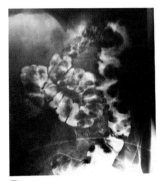
**B**

1  Describe this radiograph.

2  What is the differential diagnosis?

3  What is the commonest site of the intestine involved?

4  What other associated lesions occur?

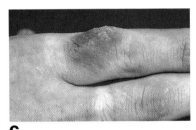
**C**

1  Describe this lesion, occurring in the owner of an aquarium shop.

2  What is the most likely diagnosis?

3  What is the causative organism?

# Answers page 163

### A

1  Adult polycystic kidney.

2  This is an autosomal dominant condition. It usually presents at 30–40 years of age and is the third commonest cause of end stage renal failure.

3  Renal failure is treated by dialysis and eventually by renal transplant with or without nephrectomy if the large kidneys are causing symptoms, e.g. pain or infection. As this is an autosomal dominant condition, genetic counselling is also needed.

### B

1  Barium enema showing multiple gas-filled colonic cysts (1–2 cm in diameter): pneumatosis coli.

2  Multiple polyposis, cystic lymphangioma, hydatid cysts.

3  May occur at any point of the small and large intestine but most commonly in the jejunum.

4  Obstructive airways disease, enteritis, diverticulitis and following colonoscopy.

### C

1  Soft, red erythematous nodular lesion on the finger.

2  Fish tank granuloma.

3  Atypical mycobacterium.

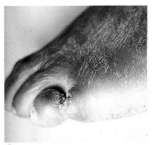

**A**

1 Describe this lesion.
2 What is it called?
3 What are the pathological changes?

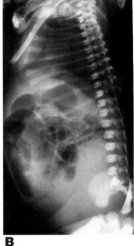

**B**

1 What does this radiograph show?
2 What are the possible causes of this condition?
3 What causes a meconium ileus?

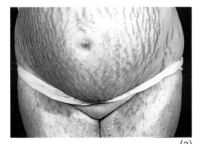

(a)

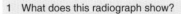

**C** (b)

1 What do these figures show?
2 What is the causative factor in (a)?

# Answers page 165

## A

1 Fibrous stricture that encircles the little toe at the level of the metatarsophalangeal joint, leading eventually to spontaneous amputation.

2 Ainhum (little toe autoamputation).

3 It may be attributable to abnormal fibrogenesis, with the overproduction of fibrous tissue in response to multiple infection in Africans who habitually walk with bare feet. Obstruction of the posterior tibial artery, together with angiodysplasia of the plantar arterial arch and its branches, have been demonstrated in some cases.

## B

1 Neonatal intestinal obstruction.

2 Duodenal atresia, duodenal bands, annular pancreas, Ladd's bands, midgut volvulus, meconium ileus, strangulated hernia.

3 Meconium ileus is found in children with cystic fibrosis, which affects pancreatic secretions and causes meconium to become inspissated, leading to blockage of the ileum.

## C

1 Cutaneous stretch marks: (a) striae gravidarum; (b) skin marks following acute pancreatitis.

2 Pregnancy.

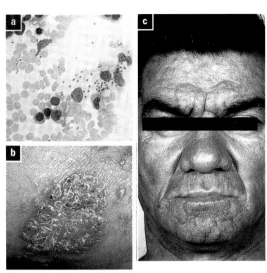

1 What are these lesions?
2 What are the causes?
3 What is the method of transmission?

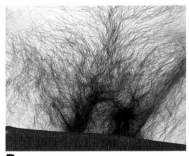

1 What is the most likely cause of this painless swelling in a 32-year-old male, occurring five years after surgical amputation of the ipsilateral great toe?
2 What is the differential diagnosis of this swelling?
3 How would you differentiate clinically between a palpable lymph node and an ectopic testis?

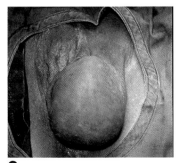

1 Describe this lesion of the vulva.
2 What are the differential diagnoses?

# Answers page 167

### A

1  Old World cutaneous leishmaniasis.

2  *Leishmania tropica, Leishmania major* and *Leishmania aethiopica.*

3  Sandfly bite.

### B

1  Malignant lymph node secondary to a malignant melanoma.

2  The differential diagnoses of a swelling in the inguinal region are: femoral and inguinal herniae; an enlarged lymph node; saphenovarix; ectopic testis; psoas abscess or bursa; femoral aneurysm; lipoma; hydrocele of a femoral hernial sac.

3  The underdeveloped and empty scrotum, together with a palpable swelling along the line of migration of the testis suggest an ectopic testis.

### C

1  Pedunculated, oval mass with normal overlying skin.

2  Bartholin cyst, Bartholin's abscess, sebaceous cyst, subcutaneous tumour such as benign or malignant lipomas, fibromas, neurofibromas, leiomyomas and vascular lesions.

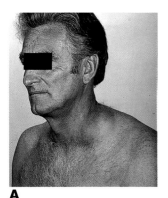

**A**

1  Describe the cervical abnormality in this figure.

2  What is the differential diagnosis?

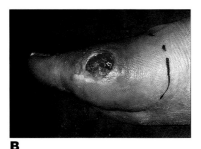

**B**

1  This is an ulcer over the first metatarsophalangeal joint in a diabetic patient. Why are diabetic patients particularly prone to ulcers?

2  What neuropathic changes occur in the diabetic foot?

3  How should the diabetic patient be managed in order to decrease problems with the diabetic foot?

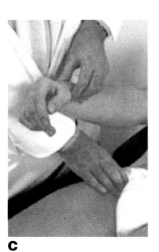

**C**

This patient presented with a high brachial blood pressure.

1  Describe the abnormal sign being demonstrated.

2  What is the suspected diagnosis?

3  What abnormalities may be found on a chest radiograph?

# Answers page 169

## A

1  A bosselated swelling at the root of the neck. On examination it was soft, fluctuant and transilluminated; at operation it was found to be a lipoma.

2  The commonest lump in the neck is a lymph node, usually inflammatory (resulting from adjacent infection of the ear, nose and throat) but, importantly, it can be primary or secondary malignant disease. Benign and malignant tumours may develop in local tissues, such as fat, fibrous, nervous, vascular and muscle.

## B

1  They are at increased risk of developing atherosclerosis, together with alteration in the cellular and humeral inflammatory response and neuropathic changes in the distal part of the limb.

2  A sensory neuropathy gives a typical glove and stocking distribution of sensation. A motor neuropathy tends to affect the small muscles of the foot. The long tendons are unopposed and so produce a high arch and hammer toes, leading to prominent metatarsal heads and knuckles which are then prone to injury. An autonomic neuropathy produces a dry foot which is often deceptively pink owing to vasodilatation.

3  Good control of blood glucose, regular foot checks and chiropody, regular eyesight tests, advice on footwear, avoiding burns such as from the sun, hot sand or hot water bottles. Foot care at home and quick treatment of any problems that may occur to minimize the development of further complications.

## C

1  Radiofemoral delay test by simultaneous palpation of the radial and femoral arteries, the latter being attenuated.

2  Coarctation of aorta.

3  Rib notching and, in the late stages, left ventricular hypertrophy.

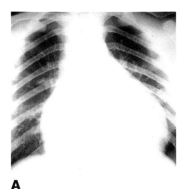

**A**

1 What does this chest radiograph show?

2 What is the cause of this appearance?

3 What clinical signs may be elicited from this patient?

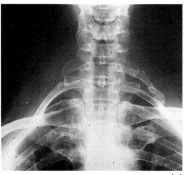

(a)

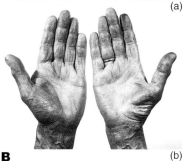

**B** (b)

1 What do these two figures show and how are they linked?

2 What are the causes of thoracic outlet syndrome?

3 What symptoms do these patients present with?

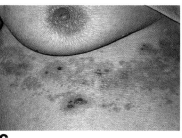

**C**

1 What is the lesion in this elderly lady, intitially admitted to a coronary care unit?

2 What was the cause of the confusion leading to her admission to CCU?

3 What are the medical causes of acute abdominal pain?

# Answers page 171

## A

1   An enlarged, globular heart, a loss of normal cardiac contour and an increased cardiothoracic ratio.

2   A pericardial effusion.

3   This patient may have a raised jugular venous pressure, with increased neck vein distension during inspiration (Kussmaul's sign). The patient may also have pulsus paradoxus, soft heart sounds and an impalpable apex beat.

## B

1   Figure (a) shows bilateral cervical ribs; figure (b) shows marked wasting of the right thenar eminence, caused by a cervical rib pressing on the T1 nerve root of the brachial plexus.

2   Other possible causes of thoracic outlet syndrome include a prominent C7 transverse process, callus from a healed fracture of the first rib or clavicle, a high or congenitally abnormal first rib, fibrous bands between C7 and T1 and the first rib, prominent bellies or aberrant pectoralis minor, scalenus anterior or scalenus medius muscles.

3   Symptoms may be divided into neurological, arterial and venous:
   (a) neurological: neurological symptoms predominate and consist of nocturnal pain and minor sensory changes which are found particularly on the medial border of the hand and forearm. Weakness sometimes occurs, which is most marked in the hand
   (b) arterial: these symptoms range from Raynaud's phenomenon to digital ischaemia (which is usually secondary to emboli arising from the post stenotic dilatation of the subclavian artery)
   (c) venous: patients may experience pain, swelling or cyanosis of the limb and subclavian vein thrombosis.

Usually the symptoms are exacerbated by an abnormal posture (especially prolonged abduction of the arm or downward traction, e.g. carrying heavy loads).

## C

1   Herpes zoster.

2   Severe pain precedes the eruption and can be mistaken for a myocardial infarction or an acute abdominal event.

3   Ischaemic heart disease, disease of the pleura, somatic nerve root disease, distal oesophageal disease, diabetic crises, porphyria, sickle cell crises, haemophilia, malaria and hyperlipidaemia.

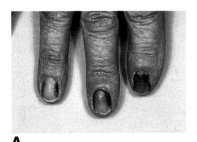

**A**

1  What is the most likely diagnosis?
2  What is the causative organism?
3  What patient groups are most commonly infected?

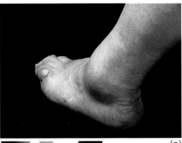

(a)

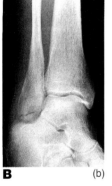

**B**    (b)

1  Describe figure (a).
2  Describe the radiology in figure (b).
3  What is the mechanism of this injury and what are the consequences if the mechanism is continuous or more severe?

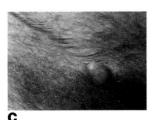

**C**

1  What is the most likely diagnosis of this swelling?
2  What is the predisposing factor?

# Answers page 173

## A

1  Candidal infection of the nails.

2  *Candida albicans* is a fungal infection.

3  Immunocompromised and debilitated patients.

## B

1  There is marked swelling of the lateral aspect of the foot.

2  Fracture of the lateral malleolus.

3  A combination of inversion and external rotation are the most common mechanisms to produce this fracture. If the mechanism is continuous there is avulsion fracture of the medial malleolus and the ankle becomes unstable. The rotating talus may push the small posterior malleolar fragment and lead to a third fracture, the combination being called a Pott's fracture.

## C

1  Hypertrophic tissue at the medial end of an inguinal hernia wound.

2  A foreign body response to a suture or other foreign material.

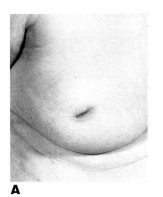

**A**

1   What does this figure show?

2   What are the common causes of this condition?

3   How would you exclude malignancy in this condition?

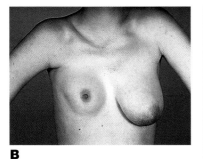

**B**

1   What anomaly is shown in this figure?

2   What is the incidence of asymmetrical breasts?

3   Name two other congenital breast anomalies.

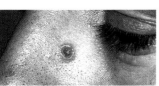

**C**

1   What is the diagnosis?

2   What are the predisposing factors to the condition?

3   How does the lesion spread?

# Answers page 175

## A

1 Nipple retraction.

2 Nipple retraction may be unilateral or bilateral and congenital or acquired during breast development. It may also be secondary to underlying disease, e.g. neoplasia.

3 The gold standard in diagnosis of breast disease is triple assessment, consisting of clinical examination, radiological investigations and cytological diagnosis made by a fine needle aspiration of a breast mass.

## B

1 Hypoplasia of the right breast.

2 Breasts are rarely symmetrical.

3 Absence of one or both breasts; breast hyperplasia.

## C

1 Basal cell carcinoma (rodent ulcer).

2 Exposure to the sun, and patients with xeroderma pigmentosa, who also have a predilection to radiotherapy scars.

3 The lesion spreads by local invasion; metastases can occur, but are very rare.

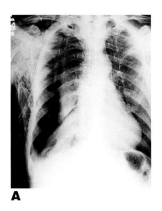

**A**

1 What is this condition?

2 What are the causes of this condition?

3 How can this be treated?

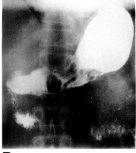

**B**

1 What does this radiograph show?

2 How is this condition classified?

3 What are the extra-intestinal signs of this disease?

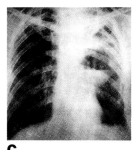

**C**

1 What are these lesions called?

2 From which tumours do these commonly arise?

3 What is the mechanism of spread?

# Answers page 177

## A

1  Surgical emphysema of the right axilla.

2  It may occur following fractured ribs, tension pneumothorax, poor chest drain insertion, injuries from major trauma, e.g. a bronchial or oesophageal tear, penetrating injury to the chest, IV cannula insertion.

3  Mild surgical emphysema can be managed conservatively and usually disperses spontaneously within two weeks. Severe surgical emphysema, particularly if associated with trauma, may compromise respiration and has to be treated by insertion of a chest drain on the affected side.

## B

1  A carcinomatous polyp of the stomach.

2  Superficial spreading; ulcerative; scirrhous and linitis plastica.

3  Peritoneal seeding (Krukenberg tumour); pelvic cul-de-sac (Blumer shelf); palpable left supraclavicular lymph node (Virchow's node; Troisier's sign).

## C

1  Cannon ball metastases or coin lesions in the right lung.

2  Renal cell carcinoma or testicular tumours.

3  The spread is venous. From the renal cell carcinoma the tumour extends into the renal vein and then into the inferior vena cava, from where emboli go to bone, brain and the lung. Renal cell carcinomas can occasionally spread along the ovarian or testicular vein to the ovary or testis. The other mechanism of spread is by direct invasion into the perinephric fat and surrounding muscle.

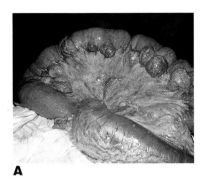

**A**

1  What does this figure show?

2  What is the pathophysiology of this disease?

3  How may this disease present?

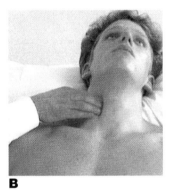

**B**

1  What examination is being undertaken?

2  What is the significance of this examination?

3  What is meant by Corrigan's sign?

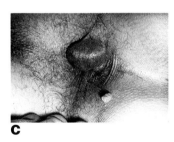

**C**

1  What does this figure show?

2  What causes this condition and how does the patient present?

3  How may this condition be treated?

## Answers page 179

### A

1 Diverticular disease of the colon.

2 Diverticular disease is thought to arise through a diet low in roughage and high in refined foods. A small volume of gut contents passes through the colon, requiring increased pressures for the passage of stool, resulting in a slitting of the gut wall and outpouching of the mucosa through the wall at sites of relative weakness.

3 (a) Asymptomatic
  (b) spasm causing chronic abdominal (mainly left iliac fossa) pain
  (c) acute diverticulitis
  (d) pericolic abscess
  (e) perforation
  (f) fistula formation
  (g) rectal bleeding
  (h) obstructions secondary to stricture and inflammation.

### B

1 Examination of the carotid pulse.

2 To identify and determine the character of the pulse; the normal pulse has a moderately rapid upstroke coinciding with left ventricular ejection.

3 It occurs when a large volume carotid pulse is visible in the neck and palpable at the wrist.

### C

1 Perianal haematoma (also termed a thrombosed external pile).

2 This is produced by thrombosis within the inferior rectal venous plexus. The lesion is usually of acute onset and extremely painful. On examination there is usually a blue tender lump visible on the anal verge. The acute pain takes four to five days to resolve: the lesion slowly fibroses, often leaving a palpable nodule.

3 In the acute phase the perianal haematoma may be evacuated under local anaesthetic or may be treated conservatively with ice and local anaesthetic topically, laxatives and analgesia.

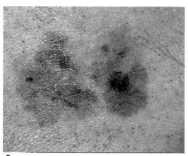

**A**

1   What is this lesion?

2   What clinical features would raise suspicion of malignant melanoma in a skin lesion?

3   What are the different types of malignant melanoma?

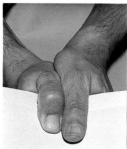

**B**

1   What does this test demonstrate?

2   What is the test called?

3   What other signs would be present?

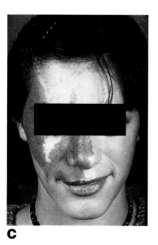

**C**

1   This is a port wine stain. What is the abnormality?

2   What other types of haemangioma are there?

3   What is Rendu–Osler–Weber–syndrome?

# Answers page 181

## A

1  Hutchinson's lentigo which is a benign condition resulting from an increased number of melanocytes within the basal layer of the epidermis. They have the potential for malignant change into superficial spreading malignant melanoma.

2  Suspicious features include a rapid change in size or shape, irregular, crusted or ulcerated surface of the skin lesion, bleeding and itching, a halo around the lesion, satellite lesions and nodal involvement in the region of drainage.

3  Superficial spreading melanoma, nodular, acral lentiginous and lentigo malignus.

## B

1  Ulnar nerve palsy.

2  Froment's test.

3  Wasting of the hypothenar muscles, wasting of forearm muscles (flattening of the inner border of the forearm) and loss of bulk of the interossei muscles.

## C

1  This is a capillary haemangioma.

2  Naevi, e.g. strawberry naevus, salmon patch; telangiectasias, e.g. in Rendu-Osler-Weber syndrome; spider naevus; Campbell de Morgan spots.

3  This is hereditary haemorrhagic telangiectasia. It is an autosomal dominant syndrome with incomplete penetrance. It is rare, occurring in 1–2 per 100 000 of the population. Tiny capillary haemangiomas develop on mucous membranes or occasionally on the skin. These can cause occult or overt haemorrhage, which will present as iron deficiency anaemia, epistaxis, haematuria, haematemesis or melaena.

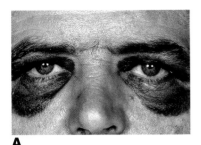

**A**

1  What does this figure show?

2  What is the most likely diagnosis?

3  What is Cushing's triad?

4  How do patients with increased intracranial pressure present clinically?

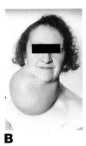

**B**

1  What does this figure show?

2  What are the indications for surgery of this lesion?

3  What are the possible complications?

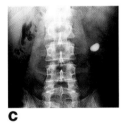

**C**

1  What is the abnormality seen in this radiograph?

2  What investigations would you perform and why?

3  What treatment options are available?

# Answers page 183

## A

1 Bilateral periorbital bruising (panda sign).

2 Anterior cranial fossa fracture.

3 Rising blood pressure, falling heart rate and periodic slow respiration owing to the medullary compression occurring with raised intracranial pressure.

4 Symptoms of increased intracranial pressure are headache and vomiting. The headache is typically worse in the morning or on bending or stooping. With continuing increasing intracranial pressure coning eventually occurs, distorting the brain stem and producing ocular motor nerve palsy. Cushing's triad also occurs.

## B

1 A large goitre.

2 Symptoms of dysphagia, dyspnoea or retrosternal extension; unacceptable apperance; failure of medical management to suppress goitre; possible malignancy, e.g. solitary cold nodule; uncontrolled thyrotoxicosis.

3 (a) Early complications – haemorrhage (usually reactionary), airway obstruction – due to laryngeal oedema, compression of airway by haematoma, tracheomalacia in cases of chronic goitre, rarely due to bilateral recurrent laryngeal nerve palsy. Thyroid crisis if thyrotoxic patient inadequately prepared, tetany secondary to parathyroid removal or bruising, hoarse voice from unilateral recurrent laryngeal nerve injury.

   (b) Late –hypothyroidism, recurrence of hyperthyroidism if inadequate operation in a toxic gland, hypoparathyroidism, keloid scar.

## C

1 There is a staghorn calculus in the left renal pelvis.

2 An intravenous urogram can be done to assess the presence of any obstruction and the anatomy of the renal tract. Serum biochemistry to assess renal function or impairment. It is also important to look at calcium, phosphate and uric acid levels to try to establish a cause for the stone formation. Twenty-four hour urine collection looking for calcium, phosphate and ureate excretion. A mid-stream urine specimen is examined to rule out the presence of infection and a radioisotope scan to assess renal function.

3 Extracorporeal shock wave lithotripsy preceded by ureteric stenting to prevent renal colic as the fragments pass down the ureter. Percutaneous nephrolithotomy can be performed and occasionally open procedures. Nephrectomy may be indicated if the patient is symptomatic and has very little renal function on the affected side.

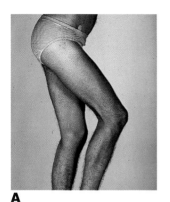

**A**

1  How do you explain this posture?
2  What is the most likely cause?
3  How do you define pus?

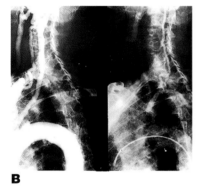

**B**

1  What do these arteriograms show; what is the condition called?
2  What is the pathophysiology of this syndrome?
3  How can it be treated?

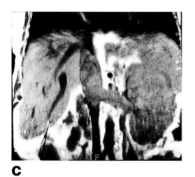

**C**

1  What does this CT scan show?
2  To where does this type of tumour spread and by what methods?
3  How does a radical nephrectomy differ from a simple nephrectomy?

# Answers page 185

## A

1 Infection of the psoas sheath and a psoas abscess may lead to spasm which causes hip flexion.

2 Pus from a vertebral infection, particularly tuberculosis. A psoas abscess may, therefore, present as a lump in the groin.

3 Pus is a fluid composed of living and dead bacteria, dead fixed and free cells and foreign material such as sutures, implants and splinters.

## B

1 There is complete occlusion of the left proximal subclavian artery, with contrast passing down the vertebral artery on the delayed film. This is called subclavian steal syndrome.

2 When the upper limb is used blood is 'stolen' from the circle of Willis by retrograde flow down the vertebral artery, leading to clouding of consciousness.

3 The subclavian artery can be revascularized by a carotico-subclavian bypass.

## C

1 Left renal cell carcinoma spreading along the renal vein and into the inferior vena cava.

2 There can be direct spread into perinephric fat and overlying muscle (psoas and quadratus lumborum). Tumour may also spread along the veins, leading to lesions in the lung, brain and bones. These are usually large solitary cannon ball lesions. Rarely, there may be spread down the left ovarian or testicular vein leading to secondaries within the ovary or testis.

3 As well as removing the kidney, the perinephric fat, Gerota's fascia and lymph nodes around the renal pedicle are removed. The adrenal gland is also removed and the ureter is ligated as far distally as possible.

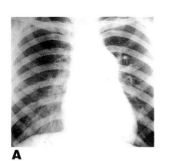

1   Describe the radiographic findings in this 17-year-old man.

2   What is the anomaly?

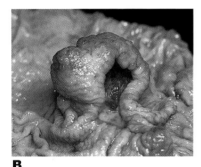

1   What is the differential diagnosis of this benign lesion of the stomach?

2   How does this lesion present?

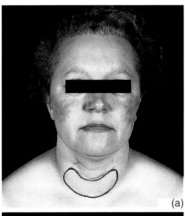

1   How are these figures related?

2   How is the disease prevented?

3   How may the child present?

# Answers page 187

## A

1  The pulmonary conus is enlarged and the aortic knuckle reduced. There are prominent pulmonary vascular markings.

2  Patent ductus arteriosus, with a patent right pulmonary artery.

## B

1  Leiomyoma.

2  (a) No symptoms if the tumour is small
   (b) if it is larger than 4 cm it compromises the blood supply of endothelium, leading to ulceration, bleeding, haematemesis, which may require emergency gastric resection. Also, malignant change, which needs distal gastrectomy.

## C

1  Both are due to hypothyroidism.

2  Thyroid function is measured in newborns as part of routine screening: thyroxine replacement is given to those found to be hypothyroid.

3  A child with hypothyroidism may present with feeding problems, respiratory difficulties, constipation, jaundice and mental retardation. The dysmorphic features may be noticed by parents, nursing staff or other associates.

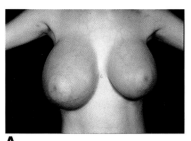

**A**

1   What is the anomaly shown in this figure?

2   How can it be differentiated from the changes that occur in pregnancy?

3   Name two other congenital breast anomalies?

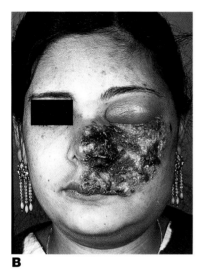

**B**

1   What are these lesions?

2   What are the clinical manifestations?

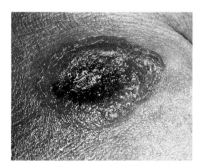

**C**

1   What is the diagnosis of this lesion in the hand of a shepherd?

2   What is the causative agent?

3   What other sites might be affected?

# Answers page 189

## A

1   Hyperplasia of the right breast.

2   In pregnancy the nipples become darker and the Montgomery tubercles enlarged.

3   Absence of one or both breasts; breast hypoplasia.

## B

1   Herpes zoster (shingles) involving the maxillary division of the trigeminal nerve.

2   Initial paresis of the affected dermatome, characteristic skin eruption of a vesicular rash, with vesicle scabs that usually resolve. Pain precedes the rash, is severe and sometimes persists for years as post-herpetic neuralgia.

## C

1   Anthrax.

2   Bacterial infection with *Bacillus anthrax*.

3   Apart from local infection, systemic involvement may follow, typically affecting the lungs, intestines and, more rarely, the meninges.

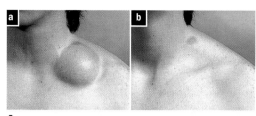

**A**

1 What do these figures show?

2 What is the physiological process producing the swelling in figure (a)?

3 What is the diagnosis?

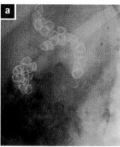
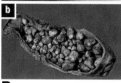

**B**

1 What does this radiograph show?

2 What is Charcot's triad and of what is it diagnostic?

3 What is Courvoisier's law and what are the exceptions?

4 What are the anatomical boundaries of Calot's triangle; what is its clinical relevance?

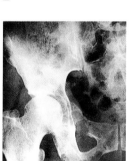

**C**

1 What injury does this figure show?

2 What kinds of tumours commonly metastasize to bone?

3 How do metastatic bone tumours commonly present?

# Answers page 191

## A

1  A domed swelling in the root of the neck and its disappearance.

2  Valsalva manoeuvre.

3  A venous malformation in the root of the neck.

## B

1  Gallstones.

2  Charcot's triad consists of right upper quadrant pain, jaundice and fever. This is diagnostic of ascending cholangitis.

3  In a jaundiced patient with a palpable gallbladder, the obstruction of the bile duct causing the jaundice is unlikely to be a stone. Exceptions to Courvoisier's law include: a stone occluding the cystic duct and a synchronous obstruction of the distal common bile duct.

4  The liver, the common hepatic duct and the cystic duct. It is clinically relevant since, during cholecystectomy, the cystic artery and its branches are found running through Calot's triangle.

## C

1  Pathological fracture of superior pubic ramus.

2  Breast, prostate, bronchus, kidney and thyroid.

3  A lump, pain or fracture of the bone; pressure on the spinal cord may lead to paraplegia.

# Index

*Please note that page references refer to figures and questions only, further information follows on answer pages*

Abdominal distension in children, 137, 139
Abdominal pain, acute: medical causes, 171
Abscess
    anal region, 39
    apical (finger), 135
    Bartholin, 131
    breast, 107
    collar-stud, 67
    definition, 33, 53
    lung, 61
    psoas, 185
    subphrenic, 131
    tooth, 141
    tuberculous, 155
Achalasia, 37
Achilles tendon rupture, 61
Acromegaly, 11
Addison's disease, 149
Ainhum, 165
Albright's syndrome, 81
Amylase, serum, 53
Anaemia, microcytic, 69
Aneurysm
    abdominal aortic, 63
    Berry, 49
Angina, 87
Anthrax, 189
Anus
    abscess, 39
    anatomy, 39, 97
    Crohn's disease, 7
    fissure, 115
    fistula, 15, 157
    imperforate, 77
    itching, 131
    tumours, 157
    warts, 143
    *see also* Haemorrhoids
Aorta
    abdominal aneurysm, 63
    coarctation, 169
Apocrinitis, 19, 37
Appendicitis, 145
Arterial disorders
    aneurysms, 49, 63
    arterial ulcers, 147
    carotid artery stenosis, 25
    coronary artery stenosis, 87
    ductus arteriosus, 187
    femoral artery stenosis, 1
    hand ischaemia, 133

intestinal ischaemia, 21
    lower leg ischaemia, 1, 27
    Raynaud's disease, 119
    subclavian steal syndrome, 185
    thoracic outlet syndrome, 171
    Volkmann's contracture, 49
Arteritis, temporal, 89
Arthritis
    rheumatoid, 115
    septic, 135
Ascaris lumbricoides, 59
Ascites, 1, 59, 67, 153, 157
Atelectasis, 35
Atrial myxoma, 93
Autoamputation, little toe, 165
Axilla, suppurative hydradenitis, 37


Balanitis xerotica obliterans, 105
Barium swallow, 3
Bartholin's abscess, 131
Bartholin's cyst, 131
Basal cell carcinoma, 175
Behçet's syndrome, 105
Berry aneurysm, 49
Bladder
    filling defect, 141
    fistula, 43
Blister, fracture, 119
Bone metastases, 69, 191
Branchial cyst, 73
Branchial fistula, 107
Breast disorders
    benign lumps, 111
    Brodie's cystosarcoma phyllodes, 73
    carcinoma, 55
        male breast, 83
        malignant ulcer, 31
        risk factors, 65
        skin changes, 65
        tissue fixity, 19, 79, 103
    congenital, 175, 189
    gynaecomastia, 133
    hyperplasia, 189
    hypoplasia, 175
    infections, 107
    mammary fistula, 7
    in men, 83, 133
    oedema, 107, 113
    Paget's disease, 147
    peau d'orange, 113

superficial phlebitis, 119
*see also* Nipple
Brodie's cystosarcoma phylloides, 73
Bruising, orbital, 17, 183
Brushfield spots, 29

Caecal volvulus, 47
Calot's triangle, 191
Cancrum oris, 75
Candida: nail infection, 173
Cannon-ball metastases, 177
Carbuncle, 3
Cardiac disorders
 atrial myxoma, 93
 calcification, 27
 cardiac enlargement, 105
 pericardial disorders, 27, 171
 subacute bacterial endocarditis, 53
Carotid body tumour, 17, 77
Carotid artery stenosis, 25
Carotid pulse, 179
Cat scratch disease, 111
Cellulitis, 151
Cervical vertebra fracture, 101
Chagas disease, 37
Chancre, 41
Chancroid, 27
Charcot's triad, 191
Circumcision: indications, 105
Clubbing, 143, 161
Coin lesions, 177
Collar-stud abscess, 67
Colles' fracture, 85
Colon
 carcinoma, 49, 177
 cysts, 163
 diverticular disease, 179
 polyp, 177
 toxic megacolon, 75
Condylomata accuminata, 143
Corneal calcification, 109
Coronary artery stenosis, 87
Corrigan's sign, 179
Courvoisier's Law, 191
Crohn's disease, 5, 7
 extra-intestinal manifestations, 129, 161
Cullen's sign, 53
Cushing's triad, 183
Cystic hygroma, 103
Cysts
 Bartholin's, 131
 branchial, 73
 colon, 163
 oral/facial, 51
 thyroglossal, 13, 45, 81

Dehydration in babies, 89
Diabetes mellitus, 169

Diaphragmatic hernia, 77
Dinner fork deformity, 85
Dislocation, shoulder, 11
Disseminated intravascular coagulation,
 127
Diverticular disease, 179
Down's syndrome, 29
Dracunculus medinensis, 113
Ductus arteriosus, patent, 187
Duodenal ulcer, 5
Dysphagia, sideropenic, 31

Eczema of the nipple, 147
Elephantiasis, 95, 135
Emboli, septic, 53
Emphysema, surgical, 177
Endocarditis, subacute bacterial, 53
Enteritis, tuberculous, 85
Episcleritis, 161
Erysipelas, 151
Erysipeloid infection, 109
Erythema, palmar, 143
Erythema ab igne, 9
Erythema nodosum, 161
Ethmoid fibrous dysplasia, 81
Exomphalos, 5
Eye,
 acute glaucoma, 57
 corneal calcification, 109
 inflammatory bowel disease, 161
 orbital bruising, 17, 183

Facial deformity, 3
Facial fractures, 19, 47
Fatty apron, 31
Femoral artery stenosis, 1
Femur fractures, 69, 117
Fibroma, umbilical, 121
Filariasis, 95, 135
Finger: infections 45, 101, 141, 173
Fish tank granuloma, 163
Fissure, anal, 115
Fistula
 in ano, 15, 157
 branchial, 107
 mammary, 7
 tracheal, 89
 urachal, 23
 vesicocolic, 43
Fleas, 117
Fluid thrill, 1
Folliculitis, 71
Foreign body granuloma, 139
Fracture blister, 119
Fractures
 comminuted, 155
 greenstick, 153, 155

impacted, 155
*see also specific bones*
Froment's test, 181
Frontal sinus
  mucocele, 51
  sinusitis, 93
Fungal skin infections, 33, 145
  Madura foot, 123

Galactorrhoea, 121, 125
Gallstones, 191
Gangrene
  foot, 11
  gas, 85
  hand, 21, 35
  synergistic, 47
Gastric disorders *see* Stomach
Gigantism of individual limb, 103
Glaucoma, acute, 57
Glomus tumour, 71
Goitre, 35, 127, 183
Goodsall's rule, 15, 157
Granuloma
  fish tank, 163
  foreign body, 139
  Stewart's lethal midline, 3
Greenstick fracture, 153
Grey Turner's sign, 147
Guinea worm, 113
Gynaecomastia, 133

Haemangioma, 181
Haematoma
  facial, 119
  perianal, 179
Haemorrhoids
  strangulated, 29
  third degree, 39
  thrombosed external pile, 179
Hand infections, 43, 45, 109, 135
  lymphangitis, 37
  paronychia, 101, 141
Heart,
  surface markings, 87
  *see also* Cardiac disorders
Hepatosplenomegaly, 67, 127
Hernia
  diaphragmatic, 77
  due to ascites, 157
  femoral, 1, 13
  hiatus, 65
  incisional, 17, 83
  inguinal, 1, 129
  para-umbilical, 101
  strangulation, 13
  umbilical, 101

Herpes zoster, 171, 189
Herpetic whitlow, 43
Hiatus hernia, 65
Hirschsprung's disease, 99
Hodgkin's lymphoma, 75
Humerus fracture, 111
Hutchinson's lentigo, 181
Hydatid lung abscess, 61
Hydradenitis, suppurative, 19, 37
Hygroma, cystic, 103
Hypercalcaemia, 109
Hypertelorism, 3
Hypocalcaemia, 67
Hypospadias, 121
Hypothyroidism, 187

Ileostomy, 55
Inflammation, chronic: causes, 13, 33
Inflammatory bowel disease, 5
  Crohn's disease, 5, 7
  extra-intestinal manifestations, 129, 161
  medical treatment, 129
  ulcerative colitis, 75, 161
Insect bites, 59
Intestinal disorders
  caecal volvulus, 47
  ileostomy, 55
  intestinal ischaemia, 21
  in neonates, 5, 23, 99, 161, 165
  tuberculous enteritis, 85
  *see also* Colon; Inflammatory bowel
    disease
Intracranial pressure, increased, 183
Intussusception, 161
Ischaemia
  cardiac, 87
  hand, 133
  intestinal, 21
  lower leg, 1, 27
  Volkmann's contracture, 49
Itch mite, 137

Jaundice, 123

Keloid scar, 95
Knee,
  dislocation, 137
  rheumatoid arthritis, 115

Larvae migrans, cutaneous, 113
Le Fort lines, 18
Leiomyoma
  abdominal wall, 115
  stomach, 187
Leishmaniasis (cutaneous), 167
Leprosy, 149
Leriche's syndrome, 1
Lice, head, 9

Lichen sclerosis et atrophicus, 105
Lip: Crohn's disease, 161
Lipodermatosclerosis, 147
Lipoma
  abdominal wall, 115
  neck, 169
Liver disorders, 67, 127, 143
Lung,
  abscess, 61
  metastases, 177
Lymph nodes, neck distribution, 19
Lymphadenopathy
  causes, 19
  cervical, 87
  degenerative, 67
  inguinal, 111
    differential diagnosis, 167
  suppurative, 69
  supraclavicular, 87
Lymphangitis, 37
Lymphoedema, 103, 135
Lymphoma, 25
  Hodgkin's, 75

Madura foot, 123
Malaria, 161
Malleolus, lateral: fracture, 173
Marjolin's ulcer, 109, 147
Maxilla
  fibrous dysplasia, 81
  fracture, 17
Meckel's diverticulum, 99
Meconium ileus, 24, 165
Meconium peritonitis, 139
Megacolon, toxic, 75
Melanoma, malignant, 55, 83, 157, 181
Metastases,
  bone, 69
  cannon-ball, 177
Micrognathia, 81
Milian's ear sign, 151
Mondor's disease, 119
Mosquito, anopheles, 161
Mucocele, frontal sinus, 51
Mumps, 57
Myxoma, atrial, 93

Naevus, 55
Nail infections, 101, 141, 173
Nappy rash, 117
Neck
  anatomical regions, 17
  differential diagnosis of lumps, 169
  lymph node distribution, 19
  see also Thyroid disorders
Nephrectomy, 185
Nephroblastoma, 73

Neurofibromatosis, 107
Neurological problems
  acromegaly, 11
  diabetes, 169
  thoracic outlet syndrome, 171
  ulnar nerve palsy, 181
Nipple
  accessory, 95
  discharge, 121, 125
  eczema, 147
  retraction, 175

Oedema, 15
  breast, 107, 113
Oesophageal atresia, 89
Oesophageal carcinoma, 81
Oesophageal varices, 3
Oesophageal web, 31
Optic nerve in glaucoma, 57
Orf, 159
Osgood–Schlatter's disease, 123
Osteomyelitis, 9, 13, 71
Osteosarcoma, 125

Paget's disease (of bone), 57, 145
Paget's disease (of breast), 147
Pancreatitis, 53, 147
  stretch marks, 165
Panda sign, 183
Papillomavirus infection, 144, 151
Paracolic gutter phenomenon, 129
Paramyxovirus infection, 57
Paronychia, 101, 141
Parotid gland disorders, 57, 91, 155
Patella dislocation, 137
Patterson Kelly syndrome, 31
Peau d'orange, 113
Pelvic mass: causes, 135
Penis
  balanitis xerotica obliterans, 105
  circumcision, 105
  hypospadias, 121
  phimosis, 91
  pre-malignant conditions, 153
  squamous cell carcinoma, 153
  syphilis, 41
Peptic ulcer, 5, 129
Pericardial calcification, 27
Pericardial effusion, 171
Peritonitis, meconium, 139
Peutz-Jegher's syndrome, 63
Pharyngeal pouch, 159
Phimosis, 91
Phlebitis in breast, 119
Pigmentation
  Addison's disease, 149
  perioral, 63

Pile, external, 179
Pilonidal sinus, 61
Plasmodium falciparum, 161
Plummer-Vinson syndrome, 31, 69
Polyp
    colonic, 177
    umbilical, 23
Port wine stain, 181
Pox virus, 159
Procidentia, 41
Prostatic hypertrophy, 141
Pruritis ani, 131
Pseudomonas infection, 141
Psoas abscess, 185
Psoas sheath infection, 185
Psoriasis, 79
Pubic ramus fracture, 191
Pulp space infection, 135
Pus: definition, 185
Pyelogram, retrograde, 149
Pyloric stenosis, 79
Pyoderma gangrenosum, 47, 129

Radiofemoral delay test, 169
Radius fractures, 85, 153, 155
Rash, nappy, 117
Raynaud's phenomenon, 119
Rectum, prolapse, 139
Renal disorders
    carcinoma, 43, 185
    duplex collecting system, 149
    nephroblastoma, 73
    polycystic kidney, 163
    staghorn calculus, 183
    see also Ureter
Rendu-Osler-Weber syndrome, 181
Respiratory distress syndrome (adult), 93
Retroperitoneal fibrosis, 7
Rheumatoid arthritis, 115
Ribs, cervical, 171
Rodent ulcer, 175
Roundworms, 59, 135

Salivary gland disorders, 17, 57, 91, 99, 155
Saphenous vein thrombosis, 133
Scabies, 137
Scaphoid fracture, 91
Scapula winging, 97
Scars
    hypertrophic, 63, 173
    incisional hernia, 83
    keloid, 95
    tubercular, 155
Scrofula, 67
Scrotum, elephantiasis, 95
Septic arthritis, 135

Septic emboli, 53
Seton, 157
Shingles, 189
Shock injury, 93
Shoulder, dislocation, 11
Sialolithiasis, 99
Simmonds' test, 61
Singer's nodes, 33
Sinus, tooth abscess, 141
Sinusitis, frontal, 93
Skin cancer,
    basal cell carcinoma, 175
    melanoma, 55, 83, 157, 181
    squamous cell carcinoma, 153
Spermatocele, 129
Spider naevi, 143
Spinal cord injury, 101
Spondylolisthesis, 25
Squamous cell carcinoma, 153
Staghorn calculus, 183
Sternomastoid tumour, 65
Stomach
    gastric ulcer, 5
    leiomyoma, 187
    pyloric stenosis, 79
    volvulus, 159
Stomas, 55
Stones, ureteric, 7
Stretch marks, 165
Striae gravidarum, 165
String sign of Cantor, 5
Subclavian steal syndrome, 185
Submandibular gland, 17, 99
Syphilis, 27, 41, 45

Taenia saginatum, 21
Talipes equinovarus, 143
Tapeworms, 21, 61
Temporal arteritis, 89
Teratoma, 51
Thenar eminence wasting, 171
Thoracic outlet syndrome, 171
Thyroglossal cyst, 13, 45, 81
Thyroid disorders
    carcinoma, 39
    goitre, 35, 118, 127
    hypothyroidism, 187
    solitary nodule, 15, 113
Tinea corporis, 33
Tinea cruris, 33
Tinea pedis, 145
Toenail, ingrowing, 41
Tooth abscess, 141
Torticollis, 65
Tracheal fistula, 89
Trichobezoar, 125
Trousseau's sign, 67

Tuberculosis
  abscess, 155
  bone, 33
  enteritis, 85
Tumour markers, teratoma, 51

Ulcerative colitis
  extra-intestinal manifestations, 161
  toxic megacolon, 75
Ulcers
  arterial, 147
  Behçet's syndrome, 105
  breast, 31
  chancroid, 27
  cheek, 75
  diabetic, 169
  ischaemic, 27
  lower limb, 97, 129
  Marjolin's, 109, 147
  peptic, 5, 129
  rodent, 175
  syphilis, 41
  venous, 109, 147
  yaws, 23
Ulnar nerve palsy, 181
Umbilical disorders, 121
  fibroma, 121
  hernia, 101
  polyp, 23
Urachal fistula, 23
Ureter
  duplex, 149
  obstruction, 7
Urinary retention, 135

Vaccination against mumps, 57
Vaginal procidentia, 41
Valsalva manoeuvre, 191
Varicocele, 29
Veins
  circulation in legs, 133
  haemorrhoids, 29, 39, 179
  malformation in neck, 191
  phlebitis in breast, 119
  saphenous vein thrombosis, 133
  thoracic outlet syndrome, 171
  valve incompetence, 151
  varicose, 151
Venous ulcer, 109, 147
Vesicocolic fistula, 43
Vocal cord nodes, 33
Volkmann's ischaemic contracture, 49
Volvulus
  caecal, 47
  stomach, 158
Vulval mass: differential diagnosis, 167

Warts
  perianal, 143
  plantar, 151
Wilms' tumour, 73
Worms, 21, 59, 61, 135
Wounds,
  incisional hernia, 17, 83
  infection, 53
  tissue hypertrophy, 63, 173

Yaws, 23

Zygoma fracture, 47